Printing the Future of Medicine: 3D Printing for Personalized Drug Delivery

Mariyak

TABLE OF CONTENTS

INTRODUCTION

INTRODUCTION

The aim of this introduction is to provide an overview of additive manufacturing, which is also called 3DP. The focus will be on the description of the pharmaceutical applications, describing the different 3DP techniques, including their advantages and limitations. The fused deposition modelling™ (FDM) technique will be described in depth as it was selected in this work to develop the antibody-loaded 3D printed implantable dosage forms. The process implementation using thermosensitive specific molecules such as biological compounds (biotherapeutics) will be also discussed. Integrity and stability aspects will be considered.

I. Additive manufacturing

Industrial processes are in constant evolution due to advances in technologies. The need to produce low-cost customised objects, with high quality, represents opportunities to develop additive manufacturing processes. Currently, industry tends to reduce the cost and the time of production while taking the risk of a new development failing at a later stage [1]. Ingenious and accessible processing approaches are both needed. The pharmaceutical field is a key sector for implementing additive manufacturing processes as it faces major challenges in providing medicines as quickly as possible when market authorization is granted to a company. Additive manufacturing is based on the addition (deposition) or fusion of material layer-by-layer to build a workpiece [2]. The additive manufacturing process terminology includes several common terminologies such as 3DP, rapid prototyping or solid freeform fabrication [1,3].

The manufacturing process or workflow of a 3D-printed workpiece involves different steps to design a three-dimensional model that is ready to print (Fig. 1). To build the object, the printing equipment needs geometric information, which is provided by a Standard Tessellation Language (STL.) file. The STL. format is made of triangulated sections which define the information about each surface of the model. This STL. file is designed using computer-aided design (CAD) software. The CAD software allows modelling a 3D-design file, from the concept or idea to an object, on a computer software. Practically, the CAD file can be generated by scanning an object or using geometric shapes to produce a customized design [4]. The designed object is converted into the STL. file, which is then sliced. Indeed, the 3D printer builds the piece layer-by-layer, coordinating each layer. The "gcode" file, or machine-level instruction file, is created using slicer software. The slicing process consists of dividing the

STL. file into two-dimensional (2D) horizontal cross sections [5]. Then, the 3D model is built from the base towards the top by adding the layers consecutively in 2D. The .gcode language contains information such as the nozzle temperature, the direction of travel, the control of the axes and the infill percentage. During the process, the printer uses its own firmware to read the .gcode file and carries out the printing in a layer-wise manner [6], building the object according to the 3DP technology involved.

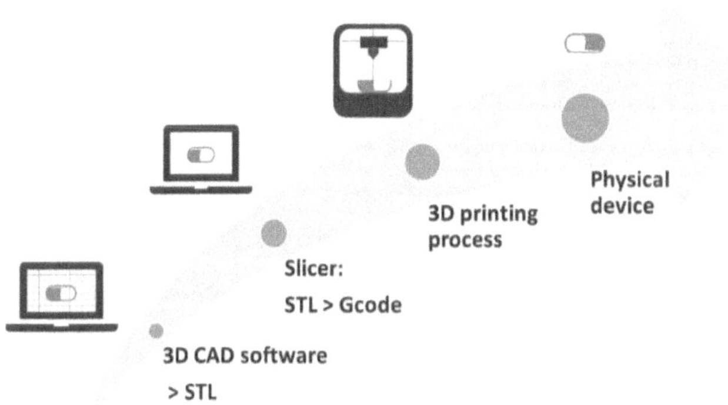

Fig. 1. Additive manufacturing workflow (adapted from [7]).

I.1 3D printing technologies in the pharmaceutical field

3DP in the pharmaceutical field offers an alternative to complement the "one-size-fits-all" approach that has been accepted so far. It introduces a new concept of dosage forms and technologies [8]. This means that 3DP is an innovative way to produce drug delivery systems (DDS) using a rapid prototyping method. Drug delivery is described as a group of technologies which allows introducing a therapeutic compound safely and specifically into the body [9,10]. DDS are formulations or devices that enable the introduction of an active pharmaceutical ingredient (API) into the body to improve the API's efficacy and safety. Such ability is made possible by controlling its rate, time and site of release [11]. The development of DDS can be a real challenge using conventional methods of production but could be less restrictive if 3DP is used. Indeed, the plethora of starting materials (e.g. solid, powder, liquid) and the versatility of its geometrical freedom may properly respond to the needs of DDS development. Furthermore, the growing interest in 3DP is widely supported by the opportunity to manufacture personalized medicines[1] or devices in a cost-effective manner [12–14]. Indeed, the flexibility to tailor 3DP DDS (e.g. dose, size, shape) could overtake the current limitations of mass production and lead medicines to be more adapted to the real needs of patients. This statement is also true for medical devices such as implants (scaffolds) or prostheses to specifically fit with the anatomy of patients [15]. The ability of 3DP to accurately control the spatial distribution of a drug in a solid dosage form may be considered as a benefit [16]. 3DP methods also allow producing small batches characterized by different compositions and parameters for a rapid screening of their final physicochemical properties.

Another benefit of the development of 3DP is its ability to produce DDS on demand and at the point of care [17]. The process allows diverse shapes to be produced. The step of design extends opportunities to increase the complexity of geometries, to modulate the dose and to potentially customize the release of a loaded drug. These considerations may be essential to enhance the bioavailability/efficacy of drugs and/or patient compliance [14,16,17].

The attractive aspects of 3DP could be enlarged to the development of DDS. For instance, similar DDS can be produced with different doses and/or release profiles from the same formulation only by modulating the dimensions or the infill percentage of the object. This ability may be very useful during preclinical investigations and first-in-human clinical trials [13]. Furthermore, the formulation aspect and the availability of a wide range of polymers could allow the development of DDS with enhanced drug solubility to enhance their bioavailability.

However, up to now, only one 3D-printed commercial product (Spritam®) has been approved by the US Food and Drug Administration (FDA). This single approval is not in phase with the dynamic spread of research by many researchers in this field. The implementation of 3DP technology in the pharmaceutical field is relatively new and needs to address some milestones. Indeed, the regulatory framework needs to be expanded to quality assurance and quality control, aspects that are missing for personalized medicine. Moreover, the main limitation is the lack of regularized 3D printer equipment that can be standardized and validated according to pharmaceutical requirements (i.e. current Good Manufacturing Practices). Overall, it seems essential to identify critical process parameters and critical quality attributes (e.g. a consistent filament diameter) of both semi-finished and finished products to build regulatory requirements

---

[1] Personalized medicine is the tailoring of the treatment to individual characteristics of each patient. It does not mean the creation of medicines or devices that fit only one patient, but focuses on a classification of individuals in a cluster (paediatric or geriatric for example) according to their susceptibility to a specific disease [17]. A short definition would be *"the use of combined knowledge (genetics or otherwise) about a person to predict disease susceptibility, disease prognosis, or treatment response and thereby improve that person's health"* [251].

[14,18–20]. However, the situation is complicated due to the wide variety of manufacturing processes, which makes it more difficult to publish universal guidelines for all 3DP technologies [12].

3DP techniques may be described in many ways according to printer specifications, the functional framework of the material, the patterning energy or the nature of the raw material [2]. A description of techniques will be given based on the state of the raw material. In the literature, methods for 3DP of drug formulations are based on solid extrusion and liquid or powder solidification [2,12,21,22]. Examples of the different 3DP technologies and a schematic representation of some printed devices are given in Figure 2.

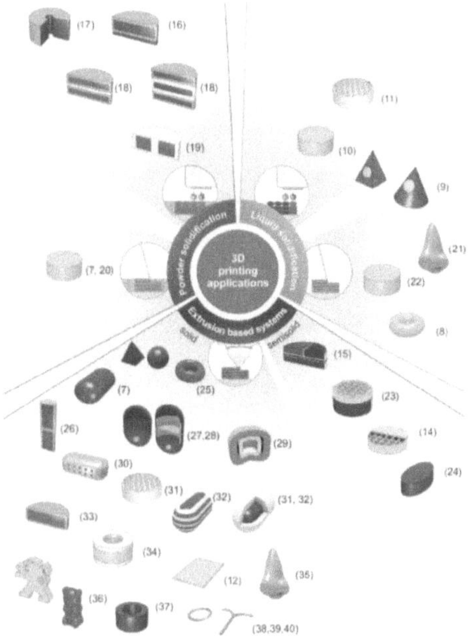

Fig. 2. Examples of printed DDS, associated to their printing techniques [12].

I.1.1   Technologies based on powder solidification

I.1.1.1   Drop-on-solid deposition

Techniques based on powder solidification were the first to be investigated and described in the field of pharmaceutics. The process is carried out following the desktop inkjet printer model and is named "drop-on-solid deposition" (DOS), also known as the Theriform™ process [1]. In such systems, droplets of ink are sprayed onto a powder bed from the print head to create part layers (Fig. 3). The ink forms a continuous pattern that solidifies and allows the adjacent layers of the printed material to hold together, generating a 2D pattern. Between each step, the formed object is lowered, free powder is spread by a roller and the process may continue. The geometry is created by stacking agglomerated layers in sequence to achieve a 3D structure [23]. The solidification step is similar to the wet granulation process as the ink acts as a binder to form a bridge between particles or to dissolve them to promote their recrystallization [22]. This method is described as fast and efficient [24]. DOS offers the possibility to develop DDS with microstructures that can control the release profiles of a loaded drug.

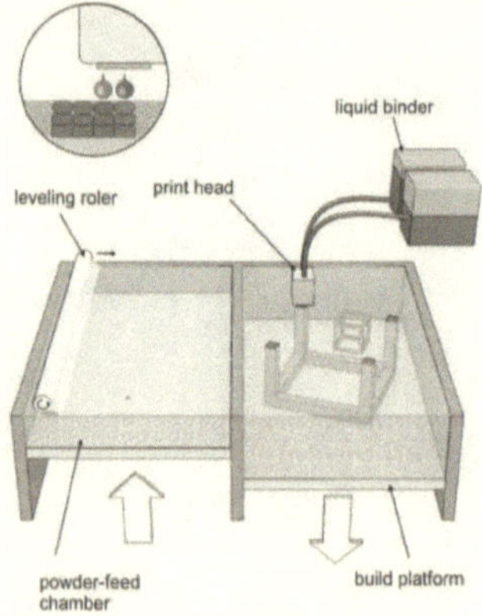

Fig. 3. Schematic representation of DOS technique [12].

The first 3D-printed tablet (Spritam®) approved by the US FDA was developed by Aprecia Pharmaceuticals. ZipDose® technology was used to print their dosage form based on the DOS technique but adapted to large-scale production [12]. Briefly, the drug particles are spread onto a thin layer of powder. The technology uses a selective jetting mode to bind particles together and create a porous surface. Then, this process is repeated to build the dosage form layer-by-layer. Spritam® is a fast-disintegrating dosage form that includes a high dose of levetiracetam (up to 1 g) and that is able to overcome swallowing difficulties in patients with swallowing impairments [1,25].

I.1.1.2 Selective laser sintering

This technique is similar to that based on DOS but, in this case, ink is not used as a binder. Selective laser sintering is carried out by a print head that is able to generate a high-energy beam [12] that solidifies the layers in the powder bed using heat from the laser beam. The melting step (or sintering) is performed just below the melting temperature (Fig. 4). In comparison with devices made using DOS, the porosity is reduced and selective laser sintering allows the printing of denser DDS [24]. Fina et al. developed an acetaminophen orodispersible tablet using two kinds of thermoplastic polymers, namely Kollicoat® IR (75% polyvinyl alcohol and 25% polyethylene glycol copolymer) and Eudragit® L100-55 (50% methacrylic acid and 50% ethyl acrylate copolymer) [26]. The main advantage of this technique is its ability to create high-quality objects that are characterized by a very high resolution. However, degradation may appear in the objects due to their exposure to the laser beam.

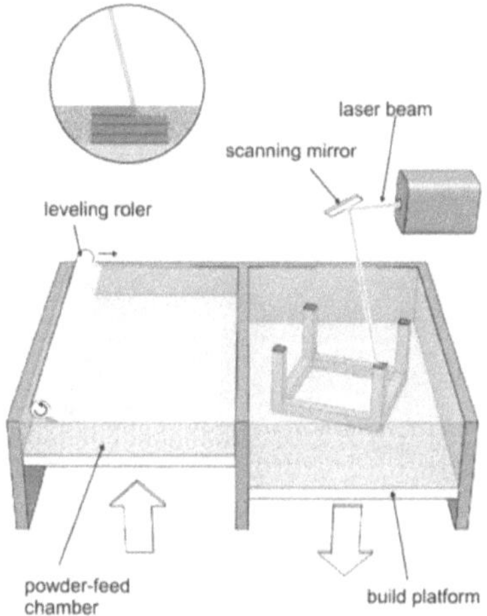

Fig. 4. Schematic representation of selective laser sintering technique [12].

I.1.2 Technologies based on liquid solidification

I.1.2.1 Drop-on-drop deposition

In this case, the object is built using droplets of ink that are deposited layer-wise and cured either by air cooling or high-energy light. Drop-on-drop deposition (DOD) technology is similar to the aforementioned DOS but, in this process, no powder bed is required (Fig. 5). However, the ink must be loaded with both drug and excipient(s). In this technology, the print heads generate the droplets using either a piezoelectric crystal or a thermal element. In DOD, the printer may be equipped with a print head that has an ink reservoir and multiple channel nozzles [22]. The piezoelectric print head applies an electric current by way of a transducer to modify the shape or size of the crystal and causes the liquid to flow from the nozzle. The thermal print head applies an electric current using a film resistor to generate heat that will create a vapour bubble. The expansion of the bubble inside the chamber allows droplets of ink to be ejected [27]. Therefore, the key parameters are the viscosity and the surface tension of the ink [16].

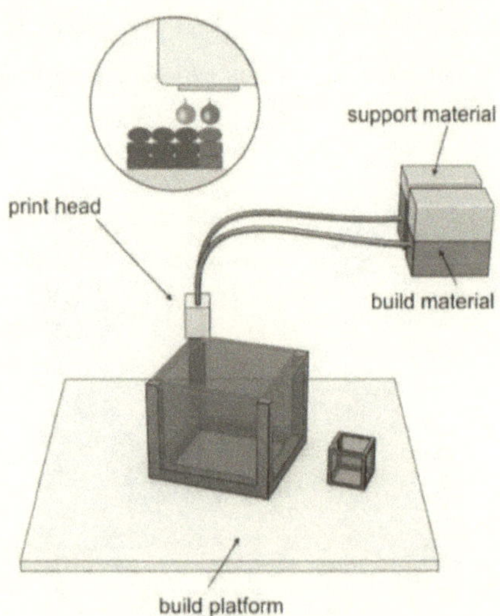

Fig. 5. Schematic representation of DOD deposition technique [12].

In the pharmaceutical field, DOD technology has been investigated to create modified-release dosage forms using molten wax. Kyobula et al. used this technique to print solid tablets from beeswax droplets loaded with fenofibrate [28]. Moreover, 3D printed products can reach a microscopic scale due to the high resolution provided by the DOD technique [1]. However, the process can be challenging to implement as a balance must be found between the jetting properties and the rapid solidification. The geometries of each object are highly dependent on droplet behaviours such as the flight pathway, wettability and impaction onto the surface of the build platform [20].

I.1.2.2   Stereolithography

Stereolithography or photopolymerization is based on a liquid resin that is held in a vat and cured by ultraviolet (UV) light or a high-energy light source. Polymerization (e.g. cross-linking) between monomers is selectively performed to build objects in a layer-wise manner. The laser beam emitted from the print head scans the plane surface of the curable polymer (Fig. 6). The curing is carried out using two types of photopolymerization systems, with either a free radical or an ionic reaction [29]. The advantage of using a laser beam is the ability to identify the size of a focused area more precisely. Post-processing is required to cure, polish and improve the mechanical properties of the final object [30].

The application of this technique to the pharmaceutical field seems limited as there is a lack of FDA-approved photopolymerizable resins. Polymeric or resin residues as well as the generated free radicals may induce toxicity due to the chemical reactivity of uncured material. Commonly used resins are polyacrylates and epoxy derivatives. Stereolithography has been employed and implemented in the tissue engineering area [15].

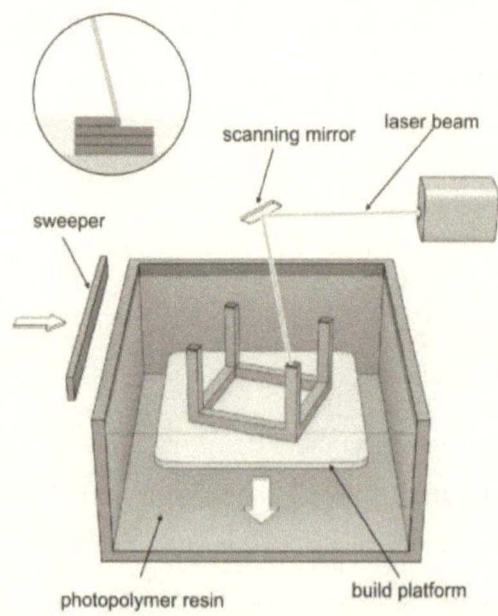

Fig. 6. Schematic representation of stereolithography technique [12].

I.1.3   Technologies based on solid material extrusion

I.1.3.1   Pressure-assisted microsyringe

Pressure-assisted microsyringe (PAM) technology involves the deposition of soft material (semi-solid or viscous) through a syringe-based print head (Fig. 7). The syringe is typically loaded with the material and the viscous or semi-liquid slurry is extruded using pneumatic pressure, a plunger or a screw [31,32]. The starting material is usually made of polymer(s) and appropriate solvent(s) to reach a suitable viscosity of the slurry. The formulation of such semisolid material must allow preventing the collapse of the 3D structure. PAM technology could be performed at room temperature, but the system can integrate a heat-exchanger to extend the potential types of raw material to be used. The latter point is interesting as thermosensitive compounds can be formulated and integrated into a DDS using PAM [9].

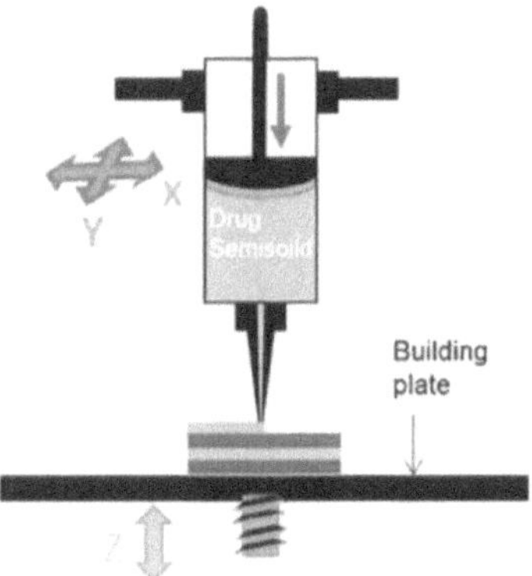

Fig. 7 Schematic representation of PAM technique [30].

As PAM is a solvent-based technique, the main disadvantage of this process is the need to perform a post-treatment (drying) to remove potential solvent residues. Therefore, instabilities or degradation could appear during the drying. Indeed, shrinkage or deformation as well as collapse of the deposited layers may occur [31]. Moreover, organic solvents are usually required to dissolve hydrophobic polymers. Regulatory systems restrict the use of solvents that are recognized as toxic, and the implementation of a plethora of analytic methods may increase the total cost of the manufacturing [1].

Polypills have been widely investigated using the PAM technique [9,33,34]. For instance, five API were added into two-compartment tablets, allowing two kinds of controlled release within the same dosage form (i.e. immediate and sustained release) (Fig. 8) [33].

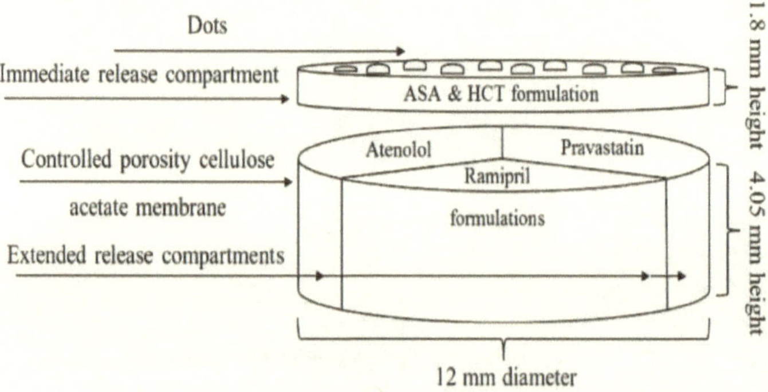

Fig. 8. Schematic illustration of the polypills with their structural arrangement [33].

I.1.3.2 Filament-based material extrusion

Filament-based material extrusion is usually referred to as fused filament fabrication, also known as FDM technology (Fig. 9). The process is based on the extrusion of thermoplastic polymer, which is driven by a gear system through a heated nozzle tip. The print head is composed of a pinch roller mechanism, a liquefier (or heater) block, a nozzle and a gantry system that manages the x-y directions. The filament is fed into and melted in the liquefier (or heater), putting the solid into a softened state. The solid part of the filament is used as a plunger to push the melt through the nozzle tip [21,35]. Once a layer of thermoplastic melt is deposited, the build platform is lowered, and the process is repeated to build the structure in a layer-wise manner. The thermoplastic material requires appropriate rheological properties. Indeed, the rheological properties depend on the nozzle diameter, the pressure drop, the feed rate and other factors such as the thermal properties of the polymeric filament (i.e. thermal conductivity, density or glass transition temperature (T_g)) [36].

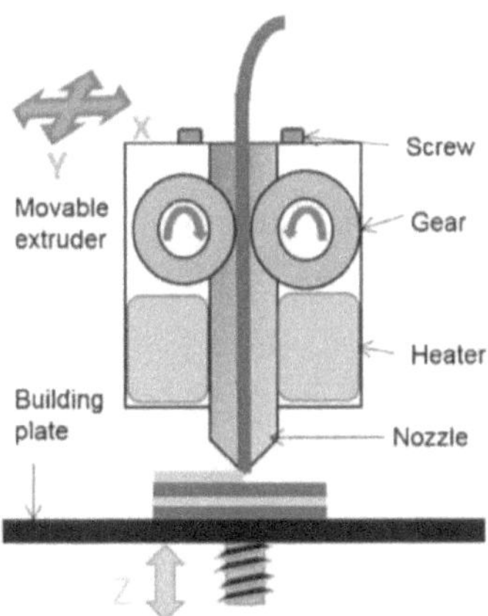

Fig. 9. Schematic representation of FDM technique [30].

FDM 3D printers are versatile, low-cost and allow quick and easy manufacture of complex structures. The mechanical strength of the printed objects as well as the ability of FDM to modify the infill percentage to control the release of a loaded drug from the printed DDS are some of the highlighted advantages of this technique. One commonly described major limitation is the use of relatively high temperatures, which may limit the use of thermosensitive API. Goyanes et al. have shown a significant thermal degradation of API (i.e. 4-Aminosalicylic acid) when polyvinyl alcohol (PVA) was printed at 210 °C [37]. In addition, another limitation of the use of FDM is the restricted number of pharmaceutical-grade thermoplastic polymers, which must be characterized by suitable viscosity properties for extrusion/printing. Further examples of FDM technology will be described in the next section, I.2.

I.1.4   Comparison of three-dimensional printing techniques

Different types of 3DP techniques were described in the previous sections. To improve understanding of these, a summary of the pros and cons of each technique is provided (Table 1).

Table 1. Comparison of three-dimensional techniques (adapted from [12,31,36])

3D printer	DOS	Selective laser sintering	DOD	Stereolithography	PAM	FDM
Principle	Powder agglomeration by liquid jetting	Powder solidification by sintering (or melting) using a laser beam	Jetting and deposition of material and solidification after cooling, solvent evaporation or UV photopolymerization	Photopolymerization of liquid resin in a vat using a high-energy laser beam or UV	Deposition of viscous and semi-liquid material using a syringe extruder and solidification	Extrusion and deposition of melted material and solidification after cooling
Material	Polymers or powders (e.g PLLA, maltitol)	Chamber of powdered material (e.g. Eudragit®)	Waxes or polymers (e.g. white beewax)	Photosensitive resin (e.g. polyacrylates and epoxy derivatives)	Semi-liquid viscous material (e.g. HPMC)	Thermoplastic polymer (e.g. polyesters)
Pros	Works continuously, Exact dosing, Compatible with commonly used excipients	High resolution, Resilience, Solvent-free method, Faster production	High resolution, Use of photosensitive polymer	High resolution, Smooth structure surface, Micro-structure manufacturing	Suitable for complex DDS, Works at room temperature, High drug loading	Low cost, Better drug uniformity, No post processing required, High drug loading
Cons	High energy expenditure and waste generation, Resilience, Post-processing required	API degradation due to high-energy laser beam, Cost	Difficult to implement, Post-processing required, Resilience	Lack of FDA-approved resins, Free radicals, Cost, Post-processing required, Long print time	Use of organic solvents, Toxicity, Loss of stability, Post-processing is required	Lack of biocompatible thermoplastic polymers, API degradation due to high temperature, Low resolution, High temperature processing

1.2 Fused deposition modelling

Within the last five years, FDM technology has represented the most investigated 3DP technique in academic research. The development of 3D-printed oral dosage forms has been particularly described, due to the ability of FDM to produce customized and tailored DDS for personalized medicines [14,38]. Indeed, the literature highlights the ability of the 3DP technique to supplement mass production using conventional manufacturing approaches. In addition, the oral route of administration is the oldest and the most commonly used, which may explain the enthusiasm for producing DDS by FDM. However, FDM (and other 3DP techniques) faces several challenges and limitations to reach large-scale production. Among these are the availability of the raw-material polymer, the resolution of the printer, which depends on the technique, and the cost. Overall, the production rate remains related to the technique and requires printers with higher efficiency. This tends to focus 3DP processes onto personalized medicine, for which pre-clinical studies are needed. Indeed, such studies would help understanding of the influence of the flexibility of the design of the dosage form as well as the formulation [1,7].

Prior to the printing session, numerous parameters need to be evaluated and set: the printing temperature, the infill pattern, the infill density, the build platform temperature, the layer thickness and the dimensions of the system [31,39–42].

The shape and the size of 3DP devices can easily be scaled using the digital model. For instance, several tablets have been designed to allow a suitable release according to the pharmacological properties of the loaded drug. At the beginning, only monolithic tablets or films were investigated. However, due to the growing interest in FDM, many other applications are now covered [14]. Goyanes et al. have designed drug-loaded 3DP tablets characterized by five different geometries (i.e. pyramid, cube, sphere, cylinder and torus) to evaluate their release properties [43]. Their work demonstrated the contribution of the surface-area-to-volume ratio on the release kinetic. The geometry can be modulated to achieve other aims. Indeed, the flexibility and the accuracy of FDM printers (e.g. size, dose) has been demonstrated with the development of dosage forms that were able to mimic the anatomy of an animal while delivering a loaded drug characterized by a narrow therapeutic index (e.g. warfarin). This study showed the ability of FDM to produce tailored DDS with a high accuracy of dose as well as of delivery [44] (Table 2).

In addition to the development of 3DP oral dosage forms, FDM can also be used to produce 3DP DDS that are designed to be administrated by both vaginal and intrauterine routes [45–47] or to target transdermal delivery (microneedle patches [48]), topical delivery (wound dressings [49,50]), intravenous delivery (catheters [51,52]) or for (bio)medical applications such as stents [53], implants [54,55] or meshes [56,57].

The development of implantable DDS has been performed to meet a patient's specific need or to increase patient compliance for the treatment of chronic diseases [54,58–60]. The versatility of FDM 3D printers allows building drug-loaded devices with customized geometry and specific dose. Such ability may potentially permit the production of personalized medicines to avoid the current "one-size-fits-all" approach. Therefore, a growing interest in the development of 3D-printed drug-loaded DDS such as implants, meshes and catheters has been shown in the literature [51,54,57].

The main advantage of 3DP implants is usually described as the limitless potential geometry that they afford. Almost any shape can be produced to fit the individual needs of each patient [54]. It has been demonstrated that implants, such as wound dressings, could be created using medical imaging to adapt their shape to the patient anatomy. For instance, 3D digital models have been generated from 3D scans to produce an anti-acne nose mask containing salicylic acid or antimicrobial-metal-loaded wound dressings for the nose or ear [49,50] (Fig. 10). These studies show the possibility of FDM to print tailored devices for individual patients by modifying the devices' size and shape as well as the type of drug.

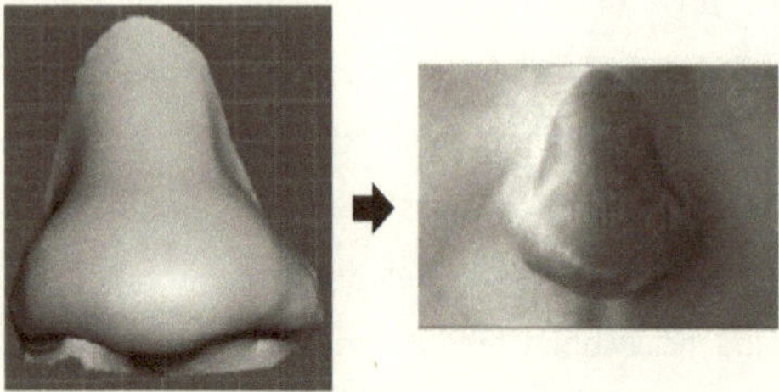

Fig. 10. 3D scan model of nose (left) and FDM-printed nose wound dressing loaded with antiacne drug (right) [50].

The inner part of the object can be modulated by changing its infill percentage. The infill is expressed as a percentage, with 0% corresponding to a hollow object while 100% is the highest density and creates a fully solid object [61] (Fig. 11).

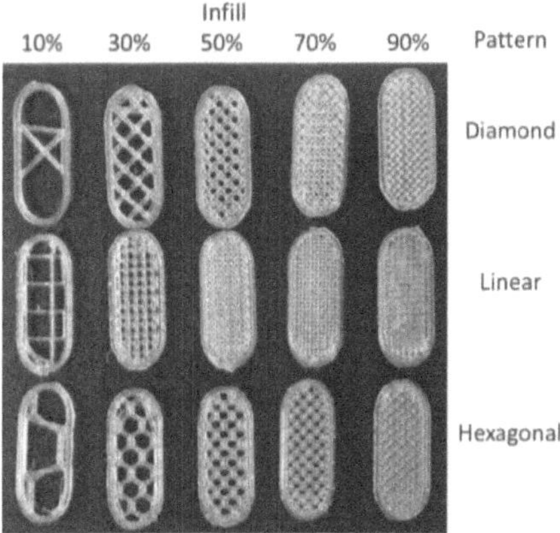

Fig. 11. Photograph of 3DP devices with varying infill densities and infill patterns.

The infill pattern can be adapted using several types of microarchitectures, such as linear, hexagonal, diamond, Moroccan star, sharkfill and catfill architectures. It has been demonstrated that the infill percentage played a major role in the drug release from 3DP tablets. Indeed, it has been shown that the release of a loaded drug was slower with an increase in the density (increase in the infill percentage) [37,62]. For example, the release of a tablet made of Hypromellose (HPMC) containing a model drug showed different patterns of release over time (Fig. 12).

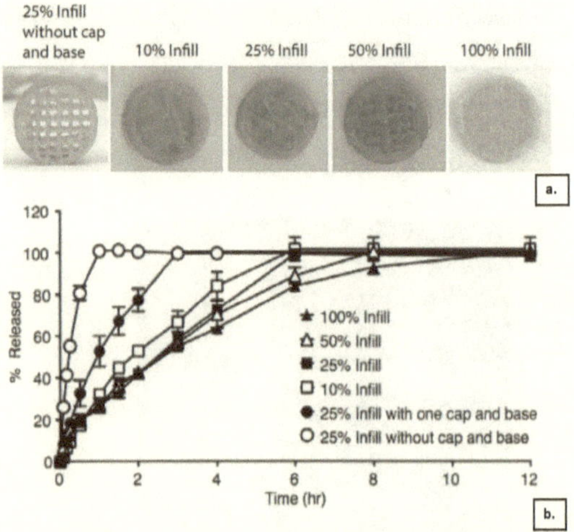

Fig. 12. Influence of infill density in percentage (**a.**) and the release patterns (**b.**) of tablet made of HPMC and loaded with a model drug [62].

In addition, Kadry et al. demonstrated the influence of the pattern on the drug release [62] (Fig. 13). The group stated that a variation of the pattern could influence the inner volume of devices. Consequently, a larger volume is generated, which promote the wettability of the tablet, and a faster dissolution was observed [62].

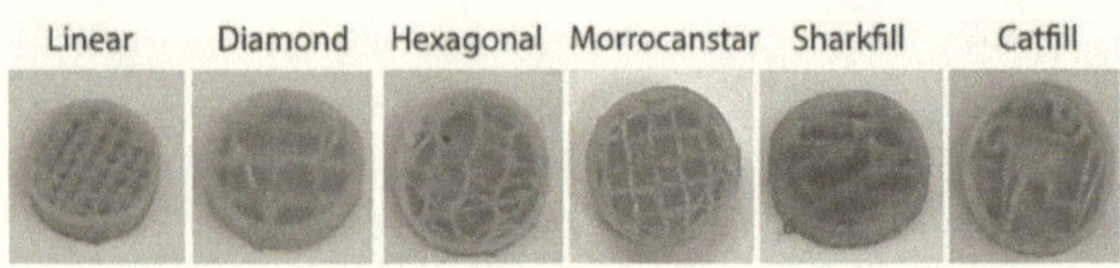

Fig. 13. Photographs of 3DP tablets with different infill patterns [62].

The appearance of the finished device may represent a real challenge for the formulator as the resolution of FDM 3D printers is not always accurate. The 3DP object resolution offered by this technique is usually defined in terms of layer thickness (i.e. height). Common layer thicknesses are ranged from 0.1 mm to 0.4 mm [1,63]. It is commonly accepted that a low resolution corresponds to the visual observation of defects and surface imperfections. It has been demonstrated that an improvement in the device's morphology was reached when a higher resolution was fixed. A higher resolution leads to a reduction in the layer thickness [30].

The deposition temperature is another parameter that could be adapted before the printing. This temperature was usually set according to the physicochemical characteristics of the thermoplastic polymer but also to the whole formulation. At the early stage of the development of FDM 3DP dosage forms, two kinds of polymer were widely used, namely PLA and PVA. Both polymers require high deposition temperatures, usually ranged between 180 °C and 220 °C. Unfortunately, such high temperatures are usually not suitable for thermolabile drugs. Indeed, it has been demonstrated that use of high temperatures may degrade an API, despite the short residence time through the nozzle (i.e. a few seconds: 3 mm^3/s) [37,42]. Besides, additives such as plasticizer may be added to the formulation. Plasticizers modify the properties of a polymeric matrix due to their low molecular weight, which allows them to insert themselves between polymer chains. Plasticizer may decrease the T_g of the polymeric matrix of the polymeric matrix, leading to an improvement in its processability. Indeed, plasticizers are able to reduce the interaction between polymer chains and to provide polymers with more molecular mobility [64,65]. Consequently, adding a plasticizer to the formulation will reduce the temperature required to produce the dosage form and allow the use of thermosensitive drugs [61].

The main approach for evaluating the suitability of API and polymers to be printed is based on thermal analysis using differential scanning calorimetry (DSC) and thermogravimetric analysis (TGA) [39,41,42]. The temperature influences the molten/softened state of the polymer, which influences the melting and solidification of the successive layers. Indeed, the molten polymer should be quickly cooled at room temperature to allow the next layer to be printed. Therefore, the structure needs to solidify within a few seconds to bear the successive layers that are added during the printing. A too low temperature may lead to poor flow or blockage in the nozzle due to a high viscosity, while a too high temperature may degrade the polymer as well as the API [42]. The ability to print the first layers of the DDS/device usually determines the ability to build the whole structure. To improve its adhesion, the build platform may be heated. Indeed, it has been demonstrated that heat allowed increasing the adhesion of the matter onto the build platform. When the build platform cannot be heated (depending on the printer model), ScotchBlue® painter's tape could be applied on the top of the platform to improve the adhesion of the first layer [41,42]. Furthermore, it has been accepted that improvement of adhesion could be promoted using a lower printing speed. Indeed, a higher printing speed induces an increase in the shear rates, which may lead to adhesion issues [66].

The physicochemical properties (e.g. T_g) of the thermoplastic polymer greatly influence the release profile of a loaded drug. It has been demonstrated that FDM is particularly effective to print 3DP DDS that are able to control the release of a drug properly [44]. Moreover, this technique is able to produce devices using pharmaceutical-grade polymers without a post-processing step [37,42]. The use of a complex polymeric matrix or a different type of polymer can play a role in the drug release. Indeed, it has been demonstrated that specific dosage forms such as floating forms [67], immediate release orodispersible films [68,69] or controlled-release tablets, implants or meshes [37,60,70] can be successfully printed using FDM 3D printers.

As FDM is based on an extrusion process, it requires a filament as the starting material. The diameter of the filaments represents a key parameter to take into consideration during development of 3DP DDS. Indeed, low-cost FDM 3D printers are usually characterized by a very low tolerance of variation in the diameter of the loaded filament. An inconsistency in the diameter may lead to either defects in the device (e.g. irregular dimension or weight) or the filament being stuck in the print head when the filament is too wide or too thin [69]. The most commonly described diameter to be used is 1.75 mm, but 3 mm may be an alternative depending on the 3DP printer model [61,71]. When the development of a 3DP DDS is targeted, the filament is usually made of a thermoplastic polymer, an API and other various excipients. As already mentioned, a major limitation to the use of this technique is the lack of pharmaceutical-grade FDA-approved polymers that are available. Furthermore, approved polymers are commonly marketed in the form of powder, pellets or granules [12].

Previously, researchers used commercially available medical-grade polymeric filaments to print their DDS. Indeed, commercial polymeric filaments made of PLA and PVA are commonly used to feed FDM 3D printers. Therefore, a soaking technique has been used to load the API onto the filament by passive diffusion. This technique required a large volume of solvent (e.g. methanolic solution) to induce the filament swelling which was mandatory to load the API. It was shown that such procedure could induce the degradation of the API, and the yield of the process was very low (i.e. 0.06% (w/w), 0.25% (w/w), 1.9% (w/w)) [37,39,41]. Moreover, solvents could also degrade the polymer or modify its physicochemical properties, and post-treatment by heat was necessary to remove residual solvent [72].

An alternative to soaking techniques was the use of raw thermoplastic polymers and drug to produce a printable filament using hot melt extrusion (HME). This technology, well-established in the pharmaceutical field, was used to blend matter and produce printable filaments. The main interest of the HME was the possibility to use other polymers than those commercially available. HME offered the possibility to make a filament of polymers such as PLA, poly-ε-caprolactone (PCL), PLGA, methacrylic polymers (Eudragit® E, L, RS, RL), cellulosic derivatives (ethyl cellulose (EC)), hydroxypropyl cellulose (HPC), HPMC, polyethylene oxide, thermoplastic polyurethanes (TPU), polyvinylpyrrolidone (PVP) or ethylene vinyl acetate (EVA) (Table 2). Furthermore, the HME process allows high loading percentages (up to 60% w/w) [73]. All these filaments required suitable mechanical behaviour (e.g. ductility, stiffness) to be fed into the print head. The combination of HME and FDM represents an opportunity to deal with a wide variety of thermoplastic materials and explains the major interest in research and development of DDS [71].

The rheological properties are also critical parameters to be considered. The viscosity of the feed material may influence the flow through the nozzle. In the case of FDM, the short residence time of the polymer and the low shear occurring in the print head mean that a higher temperature is required than that used in the HME to achieve suitable rheological properties [71]. It has been demonstrated that a printing temperature allowing a viscosity between 10 000 Pa.s and 1 000 Pa.s was acceptable to ensure processability via FDM [73]. The viscosity of the feed material could be decreased with the addition of a plasticizer and consequently, the FDM and HME temperatures might be reduced [61]. Rheological measurement may be helpful to understand the effect of the formulation on the process and to investigate the drug-polymer miscibility [66].

Table 2. Examples of forms 3D printed using FDM technology.

Selective examples of forms 3D printed using FDM technology					
Dosage form	API	Polymer	Printing temperature (°C)	Aim	Reference
Tablet	Theophylline	Eudragit® E, RS, RL HPC	140-170 160	IR and CR	[42]
Tablet	Ibuprofen	EC	170-186	SR	[74]
Tablet loaded with nanocapsule	Deflazacort	Eudragit® (RL 100) PCL	170 95	CR	[75]
Tablet	Warfarin	Eudragit® EPO	135	IR	[44]
Bi-layer tablet	Enalapril maleate and hydrochlorothiazide	Eudragit® EPO	135	IR	[76]
Tablet	Pramipexole	Eudragit® EPO	160-175	IR	[77]
Tablet	Felodipine	Eudragit® EPO / Soluplus®	150	Polymer effect on disintegration behaviour	[78]
Tablet (polypills)	Metformin and glimepiride	Eudragit® RL PVA	170 205	IR and SR	[79]
Implant (hollow cylinder)	Quinine	Eudragit® RS PCL PLA EC	155 53 164 145	CR	[54]
Intrauterine system (T-shaped) and subcutaneous rod	Indomethacin	EVA (different grades)	145-215	CR	[47]
Floating tablet	Domperidone	HPC	210	SR	[67]
Tablet	Theophylline	HPC	230	IR	[80]
Tablet	Isoniazid	HPC, HPMC, PEO, Eudragit® RS, RL, L	165-195	Personalized dosing and drug release	[81]
Tablet	Acetaminophen	HPMC	200	CR	[82]
Tablet	Diltiazem	HPMC	210-230	IR	[62]
Tablet (printlet)	Acetaminophen	Hypromellose acetate succinate (grades LG, MG, HG)	180-190	DR	[83]
Tablet	Ramipril 4-aminosalicylic acid	Kollidon® VA64 (PVP-VA) Kollidon® 12PF (PVP)	90	IR	[84]
Intrauterine system (T-shaped)	Indomethacin	PCL	100	CR	[46]
Nose or ear antimicrobial wound dressing	Zinc, copper or silver	PCL	170	Topical delivery	[50]
Vaginal ring ("O", "Y", "M" shaped)	Progesterone	PCL	195	CR	[45]
Orodispersible film	Acetaminophen or ibuprofen	PEO PVA	165 190	IR	[69]
Antimicrobial implant (disk)	Nitrofurantoin and hydroxyapatite	PLA	200	CR	[85]

Microneedles	Fluorescein	PLA	195	TD	[48]
Catheter	Gentamicin sulfate or Methotrexate	PLA	220 and 170	Localized and SR	[52]
Anti-acne nose patch/mask	Salicylic acid	PLA PCL	230 170	Topical delivery	[49]
Antimicrobial implant (disk)	Nitrofurantoin	PLA + HMPC	190-200	CR	[59]
Oral solid dosage form	Hydrochlorothiazide	PLA and PVA	220 and 200	CR	[70]
Implant	Ibuprofen	PLA and PVA and PCL coating)	170-190 (range)	SR	[55]
Tracheal stent	Triamterene	PLGA (RG 858 S)	180-220 (range)	SR	[53]
Tablet (radiator-like design)	Theophylline	Polyethylene oxide (range 100 K-900 K)	105-145	IR	[86]
Tablet	Amino salicylate (5-ASA, 4-ASA)	PVA	210	CR	[39]
Multilayer capsule or DuoCaplet	Acetaminophen and caffeine	PVA	200	IR and DR	[87]
Tablet (cube, pyramid, cylinder, sphere and torus)	Acetaminophen	PVA	180	Geometrical shape effect on drug release	[43]
Tablet	Prednisolone	PVA	210-230	ER	[41]
Caplet (capsule)	Acetaminophen or caffeine	PVA	200	Drug loading and drug composition on dissolution behaviour	[88]
Orodispersible film	Aripiprazole	PVA	190	Fast disintegration and dissolution	[68]
Tablet	Curcumin	PVA	170	CR	[72]
Hernia mesh	Ciprofloxacin HCl	PVA PP	200 190	Personalized and localized delivery	[56]
Tablet	Calcein	PVA and PVA/PLA	190	CR	[89]
Tablet	Dipyridamole or theophylline	PVP	110	IR	[63]
Shell-core tablet	Theophylline, budesonide or diclofenac sodium	PVP Eudragit® L100-55	185 85	DR	[90]
Tablet	Metformin HCl and theophylline	TPU	120 150 180	SR	[73]
Catheter	Tetracycline HCl	TPU	215	SR	[51]
Vaginal mesh implant	Levofloxacin	TPU	190	Localized and SR	[57]

(CR: controlled release, IR: immediate release, DR: delayed release, ER: extended release, SR: sustained release, TR: transdermal release).

II.   Implantable drug delivery systems

The rational approach to develop IDDS should be to enhance the safety of the treatment and to increase the compliance of patients. A sustained release of the drug allows decreasing the number of injection or administration. The drug may be delivered at a lower dose and its release profile could maintain a steady therapeutic concentration within the therapeutic window, reducing the so-called "peak and trough" effect. Moreover, IDDS may be considered as suitable alternatives to oral DDS, which are usually prone to issues such as the variability of the physiology of the gastrointestinal tract, the lack of drug bioavailability, the release duration (i.e. max. 24h), the instability of the drug in the gastrointestinal tract fluids and the difficulty to maintain a plasmatic steady state when the drug is characterized by a low plasma half-life. IDDS includes a wide range of DDS such as subcutaneous implants, vaginal and intrauterine devices, ocular and intracerebral implants [91,92].

The development of IDDS is correlated with that of new carriers (e.g. bio-erodible and biocompatible carriers), the diversity of drug compounds, the implantation techniques and implantation sites. Indeed, the development of biotherapeutics, which are sensitive molecules, as well as the non-specificity and potential toxicity of small chemical entities, has led to the development of polymeric IDDS. Finally, it is possible to remove the IDDS if there are adverse effects are observed during the treatment period [91–94].

IDDSs are categorized as passive or active systems. Passive implants may be divided into two sub-categories: non-biodegradable and biodegradable IDDs. In contrast, active systems require a source of energy. This source may be a gradient of osmotic pressure or an electromechanical system to release the drug. This chapter only focuses on the description of passive implants and the potential biodegradability of the polymer matrix.

II.1 Non-biodegradable polymers

The development of non-biodegradable DDS is mostly adapted for localized drug release. Three non-biodegradable polymers to print DDS are usually described: EVA, silicone elastomer (SE) and TPU. The major drawback of non-degradable implants is their very long residence time *in situ*, which may lead to a higher risk of infection and cosmetic defacement at the site of implantation. Moreover, removing the device may be difficult and is commonly described as painful in most cases, inducing tissue damage [94].

II.1.1 Poly(ethylene-vinyl acetate)

PEVA is a transparent thermoplastic copolymer based on ethylene and vinyl acetate monomers. The vinyl acetate monomers units are randomly repeated in the polymer backbone (Fig. 14) [95]. PEVA properties, such as crystallinity, melting temperature (T_m) and stiffness, depend on the vinyl acetate content, with a range evolving from 0% to 40% (w/w). An increase in the amount of vinyl acetate induces a decrease in the T_m, from 110-120 °C to 45-55 °C, and its crystallinity, from 50-60% to an amorphous form at 40% (w/w). These properties allow tailoring the physicochemical properties of PEVA by modifying the monomer ratio. This observation has been widely investigated in the field of DDS, and PEVA has been approved by the FDA for human use. The release of the drug from the DDS is done by diffusion through the polymeric matrix. The diffusion process is mainly influenced/modulated by the percentage of crystallinity of the PEVA [95].

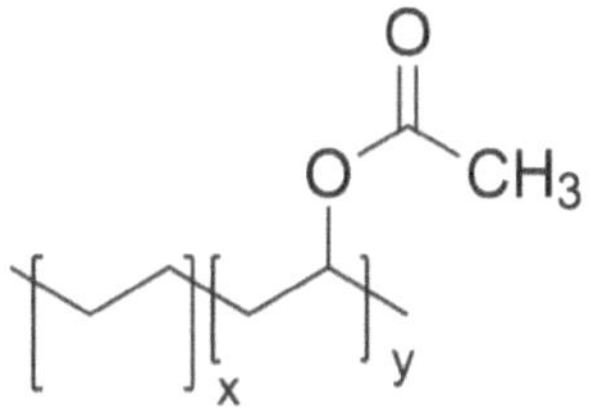

Fig. 14. Chemical structure of PEVA with (x) ethylene units and (y) vinyl acetate units (adapted from [93]).

II.1.2 Poly(siloxanes)

Poly(siloxanes) or SE are composed of alternating silicon and oxygen atoms (-Si-O-Si-) (Fig. 15). The organosilicons possess lateral organic functions such as methyl-, vinyl- or phenyl-. Pharmaceutical-grade SE are produced using poly(dimethylsiloxane) and a platinum catalyst. A hydrosilylation is required to create the three-dimensional network.

SE are thermally stable, biocompatible, possesses elastomeric properties and are approved by the FDA for subcutaneous route. The nature of the side groups determines the properties of the polymer such as its hydrophobicity. Therefore, it also influences the diffusion of a potential loaded drug through the system. The density of the SE network as well as the water uptake influence the drug release profile due to a potential modification of the swelling properties of the polymer [93,96,97].

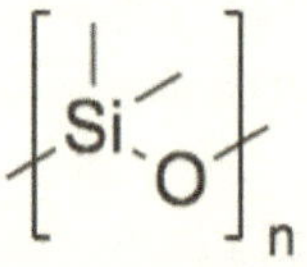

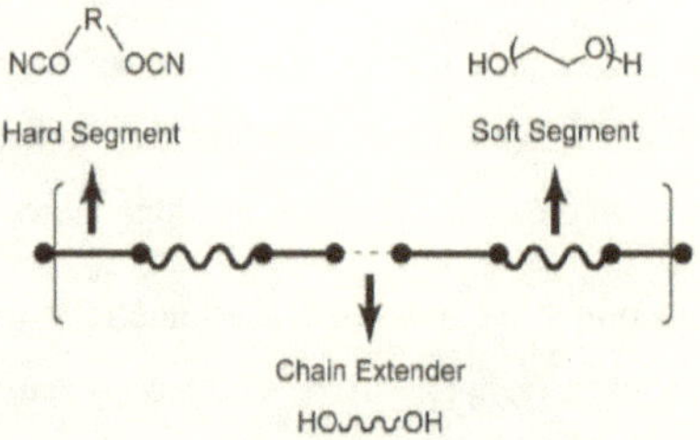

Fig. 15. Chemical structure of poly(siloxanes) (adapted from [93]).

II.1.3 Thermoplastic poly(urethanes)

TPU are linear copolymers obtained by the polyaddition of diisocyanates and polyols. The linear backbone is an alternance between hard (diisocyanates + chain extenders) and soft segments (polyols) that are non-miscible and are present in distinct phases in the resultant matrix (Fig. 16) [91]. The phase separation may be due to the high H-bonding between urethane hard segments or the crystallization of these hard segments. The ratio between hard and soft segments influences the physicochemical properties of the TPU. For example, rigid TPU are obtained with a higher ratio of hard segments, while an elastomeric TPU is promoted by a high content of soft sections [91]. Moreover, the nature of the hard section depends on the type of diisocyanate derivatives, which may be aromatic or aliphatic. Therefore, the physical properties of TPU are determined by the type of diisocyanate, polyol (i.e. polyesters, polyethers or polycarbonates) and chain extender. For instance, an aromatic diisocyanate-based TPU is more thermally stable and is characterized by higher mechanical properties but lower UV stability than an aliphatic diisocyanate-based TPU.

Fig. 16. Chemical structure of poly(urethanes) [98].

Chain extenders are structures which link hard and soft sections that are thermodynamically incompatible. For instance, chain extenders may be short diols such as 1,4-butandiol or 1,3-propanediol.

When a non-biodegradable implant is used, a second surgical intervention is necessary to remove the implant. Therefore, biodegradable TPU have also been developed in tissue engineering and drug delivery. Biodegradable TPU can be produced with the addition of polyesters (e.g. D-L-lactide, ε-caprolactone) within its chemical structure, acting as soft segment (polyols) [98].

II.2 Biodegradable polymers

Biodegradable polymers may be defined as compounds that are able to be degraded or to be resorbed by the biological system [99]. The advantage of these polymers is their ability to produce biocompatible and non-toxic degradation products that are eliminated through the metabolic pathway, without or low inflammatory events [93]. The biodegradability of the polymer is based on the presence of labile bonds such as amides, esters or anhydrides. These bonds are prone to hydrolysis and/or enzymatic degradation [96].

Natural biodegradable polymers include polysaccharides derivatives (e.g. cellulose, chitosan) or organic compounds. Synthetic polymers may be based on aliphatic polyesters, polyanhydrides and other polymers such as polyamides, polyorthoesters, polyphosphazenes, polyamidoesters and polycyanoacrylates. Among synthetic polymers, polyesters are the most currently used and studied in the field of IDDS [93,94,99].

The engineering of biodegradable polymers allows the modification of their structure as well as of their degradation properties. The synthesis of synthetic polymers is clearly established, and their structure is more reproducible than that of natural polymeric materials, where the structure could be complex and not fully predictable. Drug-loaded delivery systems, both in micro- and nanoscales, may be developed to obtain a controlled release of a drug. The controlled release of the drug may be driven by erosion of the polymeric core, by diffusion of the drug through the matrix or by a combination of both [100].

II.2.1 Properties of biodegradable polymers

II.2.1.1 Molecular weight

The molecular weight (Mw) influences the physical characteristics of the polymer such as its viscosity, T_g, crystallinity, solubility, mechanical strength and degradation rate.

The release properties of the API are influenced by the Mw of the polymer due to its entanglement. When the Mw is relatively low, the release of the loaded drug is faster than that observed from a high-Mw polymeric matrix. It has been observed that faster degradation of the polymer (e.g. PLGA) characterized by a low Mw produces oligomeric species that increase the porosity of the DDS as well as the diffusion of the drug through the matrix [101,102]. For instance, Bode et al. determined a threshold around 8 kDa which allowed the swelling of PLGA due to substantial water penetration and a massive release of drug as a consequence [103].

II.2.1.2 Crystallinity

Crystallinity or, at least, the degree of crystalline regions, influences the thermomechanical properties of the polymeric matrix. The mechanical strength, the degradation rate (i.e. biodegradation) and the drug-release properties are modulated by the crystallinity, which depends on the nature and the proportion of the monomers. In the case of homopolymers, the polymer chains may easily reorganize themselves in crystallites. The crystalline domains are separated by amorphous sections. Indeed, the crystallinity of a polymer may be defined as the balance between both crystalline and amorphous regions as a polymer never reaches a crystallinity of 100%. Therefore, a polymer is semi-crystalline or amorphous. The crystallinity is modulated by the length of chains and their orientation. A higher degree of crystallinity induces a slower drug release over time due to the low macromolecular chain mobility and the slower degradation rate. Polymer crystallinity may reduce the entrapment of a drug within the polymeric matrix. The drug is encapsulated in the amorphous region because the crystalline region acts as a barrier [104,105].

II.2.1.3 Glass transition temperature

The T_g influences the physicochemical properties of the polymer. The T_g corresponds to the range of temperature (or the temperature) at which the polymer evolves from a glassy state (vitreous state) to a viscous liquid state (rubbery state). In the glassy state, the polymer chain mobility is limited due to the high viscosity. This viscosity evolves at temperatures higher than the T_g and the mobility of the polymer chains increases. The T_g is due to the structure of the polymer and its stereochemistry, such as the flexibility or stiffness of the chains. The presence of flexible chains facilitates their mobility. Therefore, a lower amount of thermal energy is needed to promote their movement. The balance between amorphous and crystalline phases is relevant when developing DDS made of polymer because it influences both the mechanical and the release properties of the matrix [106].

II.2.1.4 Hydrophobicity

The hydrophobicity influences the solubility of polymer and therefore its degradation within the body. The solubility of the polymer is another important parameter to take into consideration for the development of biodegradable IDDS. The solubility dependents on the chemical structure and the crystallinity of the polymer. The degradation kinetic of the polymer influences the release rate of a loaded drug. Indeed, a higher hydrophobicity induces a slower polymer degradation and hence, a higher sustained release of the drug. Moreover, the hydrophobicity of the polymeric matrix decreases the diffusion of water into the system and promotes erosion only at the surface of the IDDS [105].

Both erosion of the polymer and diffusion of water into the system may be increased by the addition of hydrophilic compounds into the polymeric matrix to create a porous network. Another possibility to modulate the hydrophobicity/hydrophilicity of the IDDS is to modify the ratio of units (i.e. LA:GA) in a copolymer (e.g. PLGA 50:50 vs PLGA 85:15) [99].

II.2.1.5 Drug (loading) and additives

The amount of entrapped drug and additives (e.g. plasticizers) influences the physicochemical properties of the polymer. The polymer-drug ratio influences the rate and the duration of the release. A higher polymer-drug ratio may induce a lower release-rate and increase the time of release. However, a higher drug loading usually leads to an increased burst effect. The burst effect is the initial high-rate drug release within the first 24h of the release process of DDS. This phenomenon has been mainly triggered by several mechanisms such as surface desorption, pore diffusion and lack of diffusion front barriers, which control the diffusion [107]. The physicochemical properties of the drug, such as its chemistry or its hydrophilicity, influence its interaction with the polymer as well as its distribution into the polymer matrix [108,109].

II.2.2 Natural polymers

II.2.2.1 Cellulose

Cellulose is a semi-crystalline polysaccharide that is produced by plants. The linear structure of cellulose is composed of repeated β-D-glucopyranose units. These units are covalently linked through acetal functions between C1 carbon and an -OH group of C4 (Fig. 17). Cellulose and its derivatives have been broadly investigated and used in the pharmaceutical field for years [93]. Cellulose-based DDS are porous materials, which facilitates water uptake. Indeed, the hydration of the cellulose chains allows the swelling of the polymeric matrix. The major drawback of cellulose is its lack of thermoplasticity and its poor mechanical resistance. The functionalization of the cellulose with several chemical groups such as esters (cellulose acetate) or ethers (HPC, HPMC) allows modulating its physicochemical properties (e.g. solubility) [110].

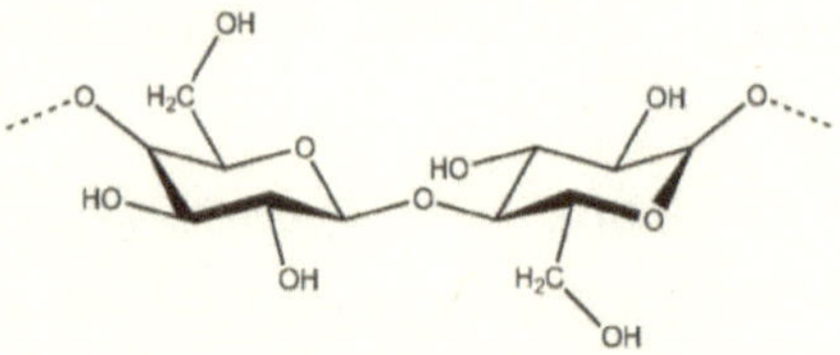

Fig. 17. Chemical structure of cellulose [93].

Cellulose acetate, a semi-natural polymer, was used for the delivery of numerous drugs (e.g. antioxidants, non-steroidal anti-inflammatory drugs) [58]. Nanocrystals of cellulose were investigated in tissue engineering as well as in the development of IDDS. Moreover, the development of DDS based on cellulose nanocrystals seems adapted for the delivery of poorly soluble API [111].

II.2.2.2 Chitosan

Chitosan derivatives are produced by the diacylation of chitin. They consist of D-glucosamine and *N*-acetyl-D-glucosamine units (Fig. 18). This cationic polysaccharide is abundant in the exoskeleton of insects and crustaceans as well as in the cell walls of fungi. Chitosan is degraded *in vivo* by lysozymes to form oligosaccharides. Its low mechanical properties and its hydrophilicity limit its use for structural support (i.e. tissue engineering). The pH-sensitive and mucoadhesive properties of chitosan have been used to develop IDDS such as microspheres or hydrogels [112–114].

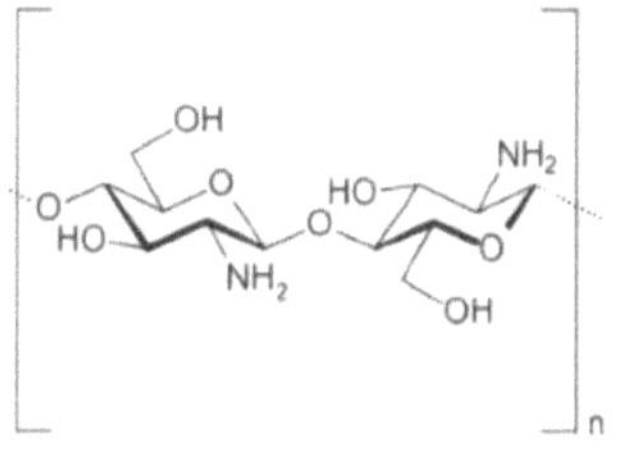

Fig. 18. Chemical structure of chitosan [93].

II.2.2.3 Silk

This polymer is naturally produced by the silkworm *Bombyx mori*, which is considered to be the largest producer. Silk is composed of a structural protein named silk fibroin. Silk fibres consist of two parallel silk fibroins that are held together by a glue-like layer of sericin proteins. The fibroin is an amphiphilic block copolymer. Structural protein is organized in β-sheet structures, where thermostability is ensured by hydrogen bonds and van der Waals interactions [115]. Silk is a semi-crystalline polymer that is characterized by very good mechanical properties. Indeed, the high tensile strength of the silk is coupled with an excellent flexibility and elasticity. These properties explain the major interest in using silk in tissue engineering to develop silk-based biomaterial (e.g. bone scaffolds). The versatility of silk is attractive for the development of DDS such as hydrogels, scaffolds, microparticles and bio-adhesive systems [115].

II.2.3 Synthetic polymers

The use of natural polymers may represent a real challenge due to the difficulty to properly control their mechanical and degradation properties. The synthesis of biodegradable polymers is interesting to produce polymers with a well-known degradation kinetic and that are able to generate degradation products which may be metabolized in the body. Moreover, the right selection of monomers tends to control the mechanical properties of the polymer such as its tensile strength and its elastic modulus. Moreover, the use of synthetic polymers presents a lower risk of immunogenicity than that of natural polymers. In addition to these advantages, their safety and efficacy have led the FDA to approve a plethora of DDS based on their use. Finally, these polymers are easy to process using commonly used industrial techniques such as compression, moulding, HME, injection moulding or solvent casting [91,100].

II.2.3.1 Aliphatic polyesters

Polyesters are polymers constituted of hydrolytically liable aliphatic ester bonds in their backbones. These polymers are widely used in medical and pharmaceutical fields due to their unique properties. The most commonly described polymers are poly(glycolic acid) (PGA), PLA, PCL and PLGA.

- **Poly(glycolic acid)**

PGA is obtained by the polymerization of a glycolic acid unit (Fig. 19). PGA is a synthetic hydrophilic and semi-crystalline polymer with a T_g ranged between 35 °C and 40 °C, a melting point higher than 200 °C and high mechanical properties. This polymer cannot be used alone due to its relatively fast degradation profile. The degradation of PGA occurs on the ester bonds to finally release, at the end of metabolization, glycine residues, which are excreted in the urine or by the Krebs cycle. The formation of acidic products during the degradation can lead to inflammation issues, which restricts the use of PGA alone. PGA has been used to produce biodegradable sutures (Dexon®) [93,116].

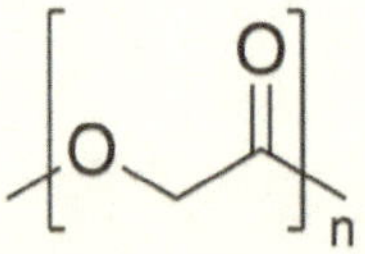

Fig. 19. Chemical structure of PGA (adapted from [100]).

- **Poly(lactic acid)**

PLA is a biodegradable and biocompatible polymer which may be obtained by the polymerization of lactic-acid units. PLA is FDA-approved for human use. PLA is a chiral polymer existing into four different forms: poly(D-lactic acid) (PDLA), poly(L-lactic acid) (PLLA), poly(D,L-lactic acid) (PDLLA) (Fig. 20) and meso-poly(lactic acid). The crystallinity of PLA depends on the stereochemistry of the lactic acid units. In the biomedical field, PLLA and PDLA are the most commonly used [100]. PLLA is a crystalline form characterized by a T_g ranged between 60 and 65 °C and a melting point of 175 °C [93]. PLLA is hydrophobic with a slow degradation rate which depends on the degree of crystallinity as the surface-area-to-volume ratio, or the porosity, depends on this.

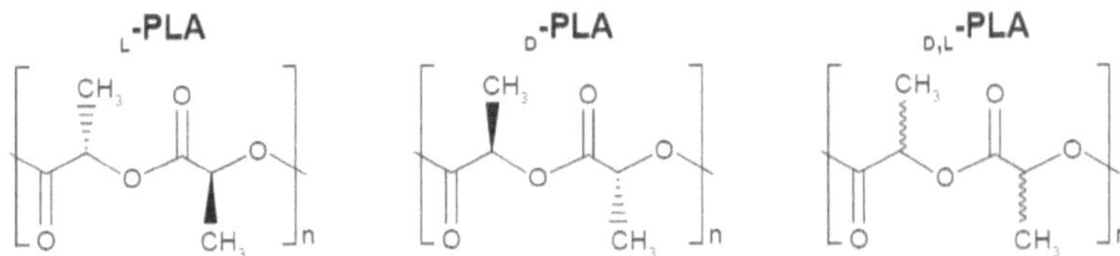

Fig. 20. Chemical structure of PLA isomers [100].

PLLA is reported to be a high mechanical-strength polymer with slow resorption, which fits with the requirements of medical implants or orthopaedic fixation devices. Moreover, PDLLA is an amorphous polymer with a T_g ranged between 55 °C and 60 °C and a low tensile strength. This derivative is suitable for DDS due to its lower mechanical strength and hence its faster degradation rate.

The hydrolysis of the ester bonds in the backbone of the polymer is the main degradation mechanism of PLA. Lactic acid and oligomers are released during the degradation. The formation of acid species catalyses the degradation rate of the PLA. Moreover, the degradability of the PLA is influenced by both pH and temperature. The lactic acid is further decomposed in water and carbon dioxide through the Krebs cycle.

- **Poly(lactic-co-glycolic acid)**

PLGA is a copolymer synthetized from a random (or block) copolymer using lactic and glycolic acids units (Fig. 21). The type of PLGA is determined by the ratio of monomers (i.e.

lactic acid (LA) and glycolic acid (GA)). The physical properties (e.g. crystallinity), the inherent viscosity and the Mw depend on the type of PLGA. The T_g of PLGA derivatives is higher than 37 °C. PLGA derivatives are FDA-approved for human use as they are biodegradable and biocompatible. Their degradation produces LA and GA. The hydrophobicity of the PLGA depends on the content of LA owing to the side methyl groups in its structure. A higher LA content increases the hydrophobicity of the polymer and leads to a slower resorption rate. The copolymer is available with ester or acid end groups and the ester-terminated PLGA is more hydrophobic. The advantage of using PLGA is the ability to modulate its degradation rate in comparison with PLA. For instance, a 50:50 ratio between LA and GA provides the highest rate of degradation (i.e. 1-2 months). Derivatives that are characterized by a LA/GA ratio of 75:25 and 85:15 are usually degraded within 4-5 months and 5-6 months, respectively [91,93,99,105].

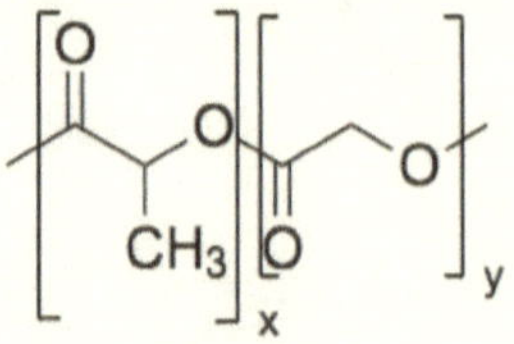

Fig. 21. Chemical structure of PLGA with (x) lactic acid units and (y) glycolic acid units (adapted from [93]).

The use of PLGA in both medical and pharmaceutical applications is widely accepted to develop DDS and to produce scaffolds in tissue engineering. PLGA have been extensively studied to develop and produce drug carriers for small chemical entities. However, they have mainly been used to encapsulate macromolecules such as proteins, peptides, DNA and RNA. For instance, Zoladex® is a PLGA-based implant containing goserelin acetate (decapeptide), which is an analogue of luteinizing hormone-releasing hormone. The goserelin acetate has been claimed to be released over 1 or 3 months [94].

- **Poly(ε-caprolactone)**

PCL is a semi-crystalline aliphatic polyester characterized by a very low T_g of -60 °C (rubbery state under physiological condition) and a T_m of 55-60 °C. PCL undergoes a hydrolytic degradation of its ester bonds, as observed with the other polyesters, but exhibits a slower degradation time of 2-4 years (Fig. 22) [100]. Its slow degradation rate is due to its hydrophobicity and crystallinity, which makes it attractive for the development of tissue-engineering scaffold [100]. PCL is highly permeable to small chemical entities characterized by a molecular weight lower than 400 Da. The molecular weight of PCL derivatives influences their degradation rate. An increase in their molecular weight tends to decrease the degradation rate. This decrease is due to the complexity of the ester bond cleavage, which is required for the formation of water-soluble oligomers and monomers. PCL degradation leads to products that are included in the Krebs cycle or that are immediately excreted by the kidneys [117].

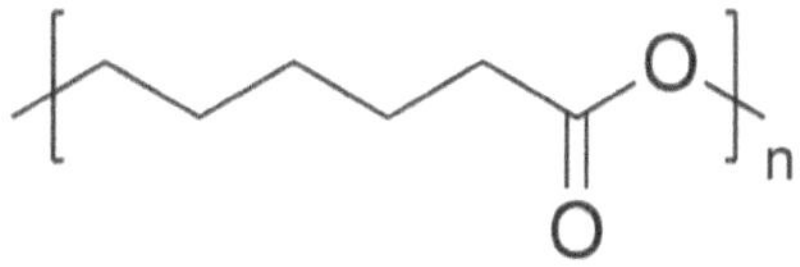

Fig. 22. Chemical structure of PCL (adapted from [100]).

PCL derivatives are characterized by good miscibility and compatibility with other polymers. PCL-based copolymers show an increased degradation rate. For instance, the addition of poly(ethylene glycol) (PEG) into the PCL backbone induces an increase in hydrophilicity, leading to a higher degradation rate [118].

II.2.3.2 Polyanhydrides

Polyanhydrides are ideal for DDS because of their high hydrophobicity, which induces surface erosion. This advantage allows a zero-order release profile from a drug-loaded DDS and a good protection of the drug against hydrolysis. Polyanhydrides are biocompatible and are degraded into diacid compounds before being eliminated from the body. The most widely used FDA-approved polyanhydride is poly[(carboxyphenoxypropane)-(sebacid acid)] (Fig. 23). It has been used for the controlled delivery of chemotherapeutics (i.e. carmustine) against brain cancer (i.e. Gliadel®) [93,100].

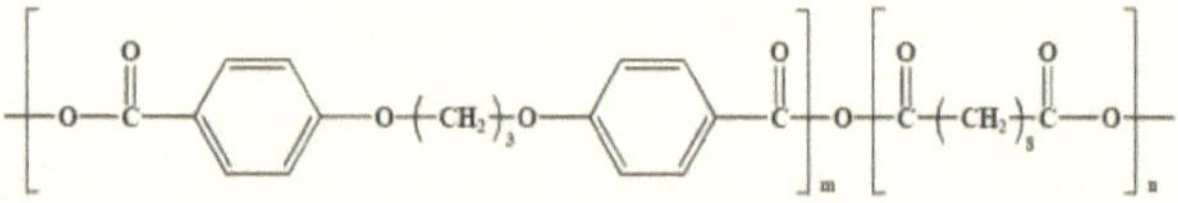

Fig. 23. Chemical structure of poly[(carboxyphenoxypropane)-(sebacid acid)] [119].

II.2.3.3 Other synthetic polymers

Biodegradable polymers are mostly represented by the previously described compounds. However, the literature describes other polymers with biodegradable and potentially interesting properties for drug delivery, such as poly(amides), poly(phosphazenes) and polyorthoesters. These polymers are used in orthopaedic implants or to form *in situ* implants. It has also been suggested that polymer hybrids using well-known biodegradable polymers seem interesting for further applications [93,100].

II.3 Mechanisms of drug release from IDDS

II.3.1 Drug release from non-biodegradable IDDS

Non-biodegradable polymers can be divided into two types of DDS: reservoir- or matrix-based systems (Fig. 24). Both systems are based on passive diffusion and adapted for long-term delivery of a loaded drug.

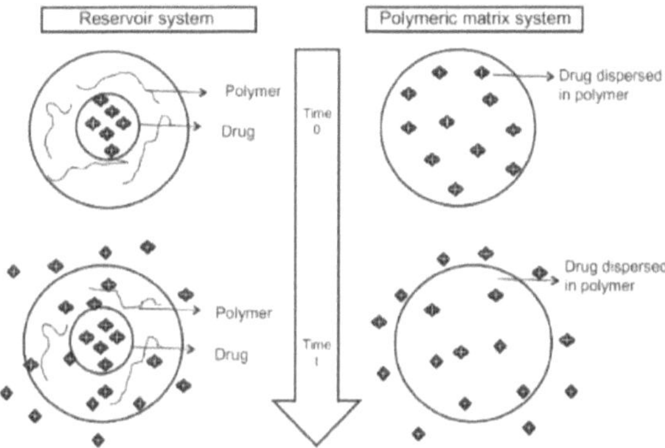

Fig. 24. Reservoir and matrix systems [94].

Reservoir-based devices are constituted by a drug compartment (i.e. drug core) and a polymer membrane which control the release of the drug over time. This membrane acts as a diffusional barrier and may potentially induce a constant release that is not dependent on the drug concentration (zero-order). The drug release depends on the thickness and the permeability of the polymeric membrane [96].

The release of the drug from matrix-based devices is mainly driven by Fickian diffusion (i.e. concentration gradient). The matrix devices are made of a polymeric matrix, where the drug is homogeneously dispersed or dissolved into the matrix. The release of the drug depends on the concentration gradient, the distance of diffusion and the degree of swelling of the polymeric matrix. Hence, the release is directly proportional to the quantity of drug within the matrix device [94].

II.3.2 Drug release from biodegradable IDDS

In the case of biodegradable IDDS, the release of the drug is performed by diffusion and erosion of the system. Indeed, biodegradable polymers are characterized by chemical bonds (e.g. ester, amide, anhydride), which may be hydrolysed. The degradation mechanisms of biodegradable polymers are either a surface erosion process or bulk degradation. Therefore, both mechanisms (diffusion and erosion) may occur simultaneously.

The surface erosion process is a degradation that occurs at the surface of the device, leading to a progressive decrease in its volume. This phenomenon occurs when the erosion rate is higher than the rate of water diffusion into the device [105,120].

In contrast, bulk degradation occurs when water penetrates the polymer bulk (polymer matrix). In this case, the phenomenon is considered as a homogeneous degradation of the whole system. The rate of erosion is slower than the rate of water penetration within the polymer matrix, which leads to its hydrolysis. Polyester degradation is mainly driven by bulk degradation. The bulk degradation is followed by an erosion process occurring when polymer fragments reach low molecular weights (e.g. 1 100 Da) [109,121].

Bulk degradation induces a drug release that may be divided into three steps: (1) a burst effect, (2) a latent phase due to the slow degradation of the polymer and (3) a fast release of the loaded drug, which corresponds to the bulk erosion of the polymer [120].

The drug release mechanism from biodegradable IDDS is a complex phenomenon which may also be influenced by elements such as polymer properties (e.g. hydrophobicity), drug loading, swelling behaviour, porosity of the polymer matrix and water solubility of the drug [103].

II.4   Examples of IDDS marketed products

As previously described, IDDS marketed products are classified according to the potential
degradability of the polymer matrix. Implantable devices are made to treat different types of
diseases, such as cancers, ocular disfunctions or central nervous system pathologies, as well as
for contraception (Table 3).

Non-biodegradable IDDS are described to be preferable for contraception due to their long-
acting capabilities. A historical example is the marketed product Norplant®, which was the first
marketed subcutaneous IDDS made of silicone, launched in the early 1990s. This IDDS was
designed as a rod-shape cylindrical device. The implantation site of the rods was determined
to be the upper arm section.

Table 3. Examples of marketed non-biodegradable IDDS (adapted from [91].

Product name	Polymer	API	Device*	Release time	Application
Norplant® (Wyeth)	SE	Levonorgestrel	6-rod 34 mm (L)	5 years	Contraception
Jadelle® (Bayer)	Poly(dimethylsiloxane)	Levonorgestrel	2-rod 43 mm (L)	5 years	Contraception
Implanon® (Merck)	EVA	Etonogestrel	Single rod 40 x 2 mm (L x D)	3 years	Contraception
Probuphine® (TitanPharma Inc.)	EVA	Buprenorphine	4-rod 26 x 2.5 mm (L x D)	6 months	Opioid addiction
Supprelin® LA (Endo Pharmaceuticals Solution Inc.)	TPU	Histrelin acetate (GnRH)	Single rod 35 mm (L)	1 year	Central precocious puberty
Estring® (Pfizer)	SE	Estradiol	Vaginal ring	90 days	Contraception
Nuvaring® (MSD)	EVA	Etonogestrel Ethynylestradiol	Vaginal ring	3 weeks	Contraception
Iluvien® (Alimera Science Inc.)	SE	Fluocinolone	Ocular implant 3.5 x 0.37 mm (L x D)	3 years	Chronic non-infectious posterior uveitis

*(L: length; D: diameter)

Marketed biodegradable IDDS are produced using PLGA copolymer derivatives and
polyanhydride. Mainly ocular treatments or chemotherapeutic agents are delivered using these
IDDS (Table 4).

Table 4. Examples of marketed biodegradable IDDS (adapted from [93]).

Product name	Polymer	Therapeutic	Device	Release time	Application
Suprefact depot® (Sanofi-Aventis)	PLGA	Buserelin	Rod	2 or 3 months	Endometriosis and uterine leiomyoma
Zoladex® (AstraZeneca)	PLGA	Goserelin acetate	Rod	1 or 3 months	Breast and prostate cancer
Ozurdex® (Allergan pharmaceuticals)	PLGA	Dexamethasone	Rod	3 months	Macular oedema following branch retinal vein occlusion or central retinal vein occlusion
Gliadel® (Arbor Pharmaceuticals)	Polyanhydride	Carmustine	Wafer	2-3 weeks	Brain cancer

II.5 Processing methods

A plethora of methods are currently available to produce IDDS. These methods are based on the use of solvents or melt processing.

II.5.1 Solvent casting

This method is based on the use of common solvents to dissolve both polymer and drug. The mixture is then cast in a mould at a suitable temperature until complete evaporation of the solvents. Depending on the shape of the mould, either film or laminar implants can be produced. The main drawback of such technique is the use of large amounts of organic solvent, which may degrade the API and may generate toxicity or unpredictable adverse effects (e.g. immunogenicity). Moreover, the evaporation of the solvent is commonly described as time-consuming. Therefore, the process seems to not be adapted for large-scale and industrial manufacture [108,122].

II.5.2 Compression moulding

This technique is based on the use of high pressures and relatively high temperatures to produce the devices. Polymers and drugs are mixed and ground before compression using moderate or high temperatures. Such techniques are described as producing devices characterized by a high porosity, which usually leads to a fast release of the loaded drug [123]. However, as they are based on solvent-free processes, they may easily be implemented in large-scale production [93].

II.5.3 Electrospinning

The electrospinning process allows the production of micro-/nanofibers. These are widely used due to their high surface-area-to-volume ratio and porosity of their surface. Electrospinning is a cost-effective, scalable method that is able to spin different polymers. The process requires three key elements: a source of high voltage, a syringe equipped with a small diameter needle and a metal plate (Fig. 25).

A charged jet of polymer solution is generated using the high voltage source. The polymer solution is released from the needle tip and the evaporation of the solvent occurs to produce the fibres, which are laid onto the metal plate. The drug is immediately encapsulated into the fibres. The process allows the production of either single fibres (monolithic device) or core-shell fibres (reservoir device), depending on the drug incorporation technique.

Blending electrospinning generates single fibres because the drug and the polymers are closely blended together. The coaxial process is based on the use of two solutions: one containing the drug, the other containing the polymers. This process produces co-electrospinning with an inner jet (drug solution) and an outer jet (polymer solution), which creates core-shell fibres. Coaxial electrospinning is very interesting for biomolecules. Emulsion electrospinning is another process, which uses an oil phase or an aqueous phase depending on the drug compound in the polymeric solution. The process can produce both single fibre or core-shell fibres, depending on the molecular weight of the drug [102,124].

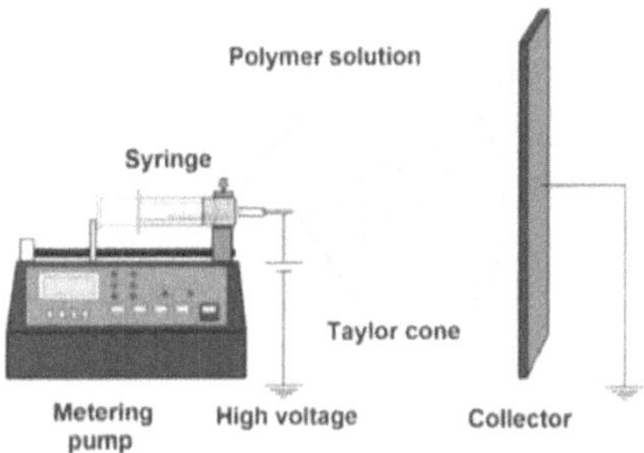

Fig. 25. Schematic representation of electrospinning (adapted from [125]).

II.5.4 Injection moulding

Injection moulding is a thermal process which requires the use of thermoplastic polymers. The polymer-drug mixture is primarily heated to plasticize the polymeric matrix, which is injected into a mould to be solidified at a lower temperature. The process may require high temperatures that can degrade the polymeric matrix or the loaded drug [8].

II.5.5 Hot melt extrusion

HME is an alternative to solvent-based methods for producing solid IDDS. The process is based on the use of heat and pressure that are applied on a soft or molten material. The polymer must be thermoplastic (e.g. aliphatic polyesters) to be processed. The extruder is constituted of a motor, a barrel, one or two screws (rotative elements) and a die that corresponds to the orifice at the end of the barrel (Fig. 26) [126]. The screws are composed of several elements which provide shear stress and improve the mixing. The material is conveyed from the feeder towards the end of the extruder by the screws. The polymer-drug mixture is heated above the T_g of the polymer(s) to reach a soften/molten state, mixed and forced through a die with a fixed diameter to produce a new product of uniform shape and density. HME is an advantageous process, promoting a high mixture level, high encapsulation efficiency (theoretically 100%) and thus, good control of the loading percentage [102,127].

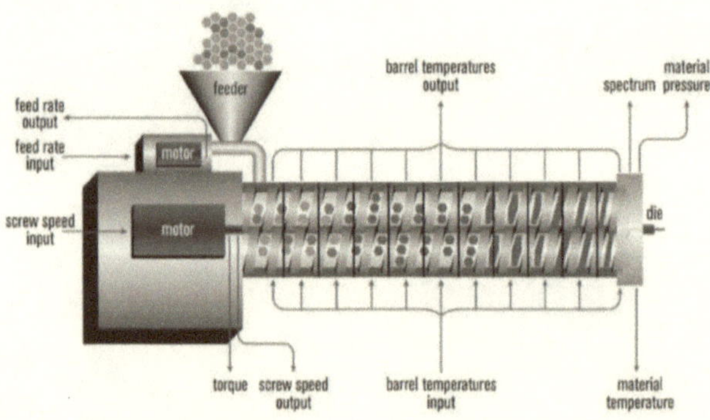

Fig. 26. Schematic representation of a hot melt extruder [126].

The use of HME to produce IDDS has already been well-discussed. IDDS marketed products such as Zoladex®, Suprefact® Depot or Implanon® are all produced using HME [94].

Despite the use of relatively high temperatures, HME has been shown to be suitable for producing protein-loaded DDS. For instance, proteins, such as bovine serum albumin (BSA), ovalbumin or lysozyme, have been encapsulated into a PLGA matrix using HME [128–130]. Melt extrusion of protein-loaded PLGA-based systems can be performed between 80 °C and 105 °C, depending on the properties of the PLGA derivatives (e.g. Mw). Proteins in solid state can be processed at higher temperatures as the T_g of the mixture protein/excipients can reach 135-185 °C. Excipients such as sugars can form rigid structures around the protein to restrict its mobility and, thus, increase its stability [102]. Solid state proteins will be described in the next section of this introduction.

Currently, the data on PLGA and proteins described in the literature mainly focus on low-cost protein models and the investigation of their stability and release profile according to the HME parameters. HME usually requires a large amount of expensive raw material and the use of thermostable API. These drawbacks may explain the lack of data on biotherapeutics in the literature [102].

Recently, viral nanoparticles have been encapsulated in a PLGA matrix using HME to avoid repeated injections and increase patient compliance. Protein-based nanoparticles are widely used as a vaccine platform. Indeed, they are easy to produce and are characterized by high thermal stability. Characterizations of viral nanoparticles after HME have shown limited aggregation at 95 °C. Further *in vivo* investigation have demonstrated that PLGA implantable devices and subcutaneous injection demonstrate a similar immunoglobulin response [127]. The development of sustained release dosage form in vaccination may be useful in case of inactivated virus, inactivated toxins or virus subunits [127]. Indeed, these vaccines required several doses of pathogen or the addition of adjuvants as they are weakly immunogenic [131]. The sustained release formulation may help to extend the time of exposure and maintain a steady concentration of the antigens in the blood circulation to develop a long-lasting humoral and a cellular response as well as an immune memory against pathogen. It was reported in the literature that antigen-loaded polymeric nanoparticles are able to deliver the antigen to antigen-presenting cells and enhance the immune response [127]. The development of PLGA implant containing these viral nanoparticles was performed to avoid the use of emulsion technique to produce nanoparticles which is known as deleterious for protein due to the solvent exposure[127].

III.   Monoclonal antibodies

III.1 Structure and generalities

Monoclonal antibodies (mAbs) are immunoglobulins (Ig), a type of glycoprotein with a Y-shaped tetramer (Fig. 27). The mAb structure is constituted of four chains with two identical heavy chains (~50 kDa) and two identical light chains (~25 kDa). They are characterized by a molecular weight around 150 kDa. The Ig chains are linked together with disulphide-bonds. These chains are composed of constant or variable regions. The variable regions (variability of amino acid sequence) contain three complementary determining regions. Complementary determining regions determine the high specificity and affinity of mAbs towards its epitope (antigen-binding site). The constant region determines the antibody isotype. Overall, an mAb is divided into three fragments: a crystallizable fragment (F_c) and two antigen-binding fragments (F_{ab}) that together constitute the quaternary structure. Constant regions of heavy chains could differ in the amino acid sequence. Therefore, immunoglobulins are divided into five classes: IgG, IgM, IgA, IgD and IgE, with heavy chains γ, μ, α, δ, ε, respectively. Moreover, two types of light chain, named κ and λ, are found in antibodies. IgGs are mainly monomeric compounds, while IgA and IgM are dimers and pentamers, respectively [132,133].

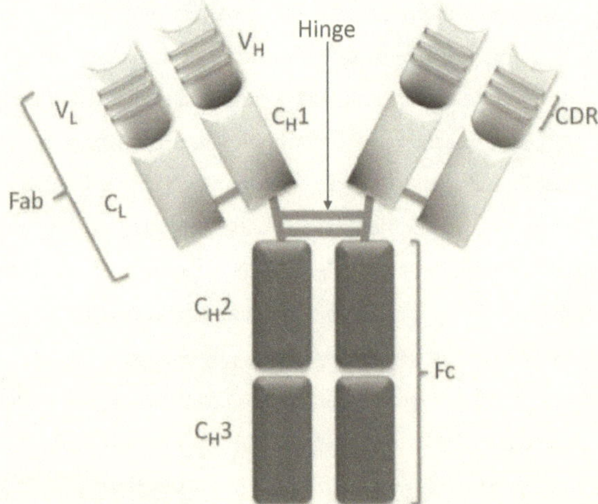

Fig. 27. IgG (mAb) typical structure, with Fc, hinge region, Fab and complementary determining regions (CDR) (adapted from [134]).

The structure of the Ig is also characterized by the presence of glycans on its F_c fragment. Typically, N-glycosylation is an enzymatic post-translational modification which leads to the addition of oligosaccharides on the heavy chain of the CH2 constant domain of the F_c on asparagine residue standing at position 297 (Fig. 28). The glycan structure is composed of a biantennary complexes were residues such as fucose, N-acetylglucosamine, galactose, mannose and sialic acid. The glycosylation of the IgG plays a main role in F_c effector function such as antibody-dependent cellular cytotoxicity or complement-dependent cytotoxicity [135]. Indeed, the alteration of the glycan composition or structure may critically impact the effector function causing conformational changes of the F_c domain. The conformational change of the Fc domain would affect the $F_c\gamma$ receptor binding [135]. N-glycans have an essential role on the stability of CH2 domain of IgGs but also on the structural stability of the protein against physicochemical instabilities [136].

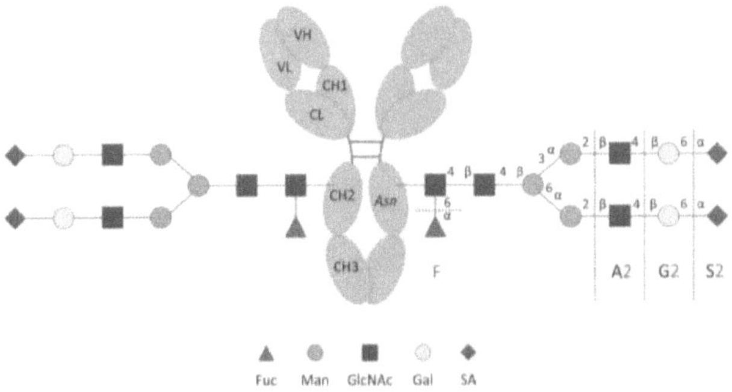

Fig. 28. Schematic IgG with the N-glycosylation of the CH2 domain. The biantennary structure is composed of several residues such as fucose (Fuc), N-acetylglucosamine (GlcNAc), mannose (Man), galactose (Gal) and sialic acid (SA) [137].

The γ-immunoglobulins, or IgG isotypes, are widely used in the therapeutic field. They can be classified into four subclasses: IgG_1, IgG_2, IgG_3, IgG_4. The difference between IgG subclasses is the number and the location of the disulphide bonds as well as the length of the hinge region [132]. IgG_1 is usually the targeted model for developing mAb because of its ability to elicit the effector function and its stability. The effector function is defined as the ability of an antibody to induce cell lysis. Cell lysis could be mediated either by the activating Fc_γ receptor of effector cells (i.e. antibody-dependent cellular cytotoxicity) or by directly fixing the complement to activate the complement cascade (i.e. complement-dependent cytotoxicity). Other subclasses, such as IgG_2 and IgG_4, can be selected if the effector function is not mandatory. However, both IgG are characterized by poor intrinsic stability. Finally, IgG_3 possesses an effector function, as does IgG_1, but both are less interesting for therapeutic purposes due to their poor stability, low half-life and allogenic polymorphism [134].

III.2 Stability of biotherapeutics

Biopharmaceutics, including mAbs, are macromolecules characterized by a 3D structure corresponding to the tertiary structure. The structural arrangement of proteins is described using four structure levels. The primary structure corresponds to the polypeptide chain, which can fold into segments such as helical, β-pleated-sheet or random coil segments. These segments constitute the secondary structure, promoted by hydrogen bonding, ionic pairing, dipole-dipole interactions. Then, the tertiary structure is built by the folding of secondary structures and their interactions through ionic bonds, hydrogen bonds, disulfide bonds, van der Waals interactions and hydrophobic interactions. The first three structures refer to a single polypeptide chain. Finally, the quaternary structure is the spatial orientation of more than one tertiary structure which is organized as subunits, and represents the functional conformation or the native form of a protein [138].

The 3D structure corresponds to the native folded state of a mAb and determines its biological/physiological activity. The folded state depends on the intra- and intermolecular interactions between amino acid side groups and their surroundings. The conformation of the mAb is important to maintain its efficacy and activity. The glycosylation of the mAb is reported to have a key role on maintaining the native folded state structure. The N-glycans have essential structural supportive function and a critical role in the stability of the CH2 domain. The presence of glycans reduce the dynamics of CH2 domain and aid in CH2 folding [135]. The deglycosylation of the mAb leads to destabilize the native conformation and increase the aggregation propensity. The folded state is in equilibrium with the unfolded state which depends on the thermodynamic stability of the macromolecule. The mAb can oscillate between many 3D conformations depending on the free energy required between folded and unfolded states and its microenvironment [138]. This equilibrium needs to be maintained to avoid instabilities. Unfortunately, mAbs are highly complex macromolecules, whose stability and function can be altered during production, formulation or storage. In many cases, instability of the mAbs can lead to immunogenicity and reduced activity. The structure of the mAb needs to be preserved to ensure its conformal stability and thus its efficacy and activity as well as safety.

There are numerous degradation mechanisms, which are usually divided into chemical and physical degradations. Both types are interconnected because one can lead to the other. For instance, a chemical degradation can be followed by a physical degradation due to the initial chemical effect [139–141].

III.2.1 Chemical degradation

Chemical modification of mAb or protein compounds is driven by irreversible modifications of residues in the mAb sequences. The chemical change occurs in the primary sequence of the protein. Chemical degradation induces a covalent modification such as oxidation, deamidation, isomerization or hydrolysis. These instabilities may occur during the production step, purification or storage. Some of them, such as oxidation or deamidation, may be reduced using suitable excipients or by controlling the stress conditions.

III.2.1.1 Deamidation and isomerization

Deamidation induces a loss of neutral amide group and is considered as a hydrolytic reaction. The deamidation process mostly occurs on asparagine and, in a lower proportion, on glutamine residues [142]. The reaction is based on a nucleophilic attack of the nitrogen atom of the residue's backbone to asparagine's side chain amide function. This step forms a cyclic succinimide intermediate (Fig. 29). At neutral or basic pH, the succinimide is spontaneously hydrolysed into either aspartic acid or its isomer [143].

It has been previously described that, at pH lower than 5, direct hydrolysis of asparagine's side chain in aspartic acid may occur [144]. The replacement of a neutral amide group by a negatively charged carboxylic acid group leads to a switch of the charge. The negative charge leads to a lower isoelectric point of the protein. This chemical degradation is a major concern if it occurs on the complementary determining regions. The binding affinity and the function of the mAb may be reduced. Moreover, this chemical degradation may promote protein aggregation [145].

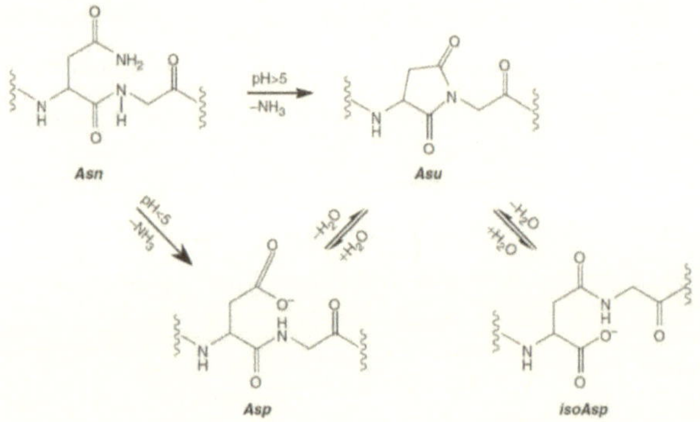

Fig. 29. Deamidation process and isomerization of asparagine residue [144]. *Asn: asparagine; Asu: cyclic succinimide intermediate; Asp: aspartic acid; *iso*-Asp: aspartic acid isomer.

III.2.1.2 Oxidation

Oxidation can occur during the production of the DDS. It may be induced by external factors such as light, peroxide, metal ions (i.e. copper, iron) and oxygen. Oxidation issues mainly appear on methionine and tryptophan residues. However, other amino acids with aromatic or sulphur side chains, such as cysteine, phenylalanine, tyrosine and His, are also susceptible to oxidation. Oxidation can lead to the formation of disulphide bonds, which can be intra- or intermolecular. The most common, and least selective, oxidant is the hydroxyl radical. The mechanism can be catalysed by metal ions or light. Metal-catalysed oxidation is based on the Fenton mechanism, which generates reactive oxygen species (i.e. superoxide, peroxide, hydroxyl radical) and modifies His or cysteine residues [139,145].

III.2.1.3 Acylation

Acylation issues between proteins (or peptide) and the polyester matrix have been described. The mechanism is based on nucleophilic attack from a primary amine of the protein onto the electrophilic carbonyl groups of PLGA ester bonds [146]. The primary amine sources are usually described as lysine residues and the N-terminal of protein (or peptide) backbones. However, acylation has also been observed on arginine residue of goserelin [147]. Acylation tends to form a protein (or peptide) that is covalently grafted with a glycolic or lactic acid unit and linked by an amide bond.

The degradation of PLGA derivatives occurs by hydrolysis of the polymer backbone, which leads to the release of acidic elements (e.g. lactic acid, glycolic acid or associated oligomers). The release of acidic species induces a decrease in the pH (acidic microclimate) of the PLGA matrix and promotes both auto-catalysis and acylation of the encapsulated biotherapeutic [148].

Ghalanbor et al. have described the influence of BSA acylation on the release of the protein over time. It was shown that BSA acylation occurred by the formation of thioester bonds between free cysteine residues of BSA and PLGA insoluble degradation products. An incomplete release of the protein was observed. However, an increase in the implant porosity may decrease the contact between the protein and PLGA, which reduces the acylation reaction [130]. The covalent addition of glycolyl or lactyl groups onto the protein may lead to a loss of affinity and activity as well as immunogenicity and toxicity issues [149].

III.2.1.4 Condensation reaction

In the literature, the most extensively described condensation reaction is the glycation of proteins and peptides. Glycation, also called Maillard browning, is a reaction between a sugar and an amine group of the protein backbone. The condensation between a reducing sugar (e.g. glucose) and an amine group (e.g. a lysine side chain) forms a Schiff's base which may rearrange its structure through an Amadori rearrangement to obtain a ketoamine product (Fig. 30). This reaction leads to a browning of the solution and a change in the protein structure. Glycation can occur in both aqueous solution and solid-state formulation, mainly during storage. Reducing sugars are usually avoided in protein formulation. However, the degradation of Suc, at high temperatures and acidic pH, causes hydrolysis issues. Suc is a disaccharide composed of glucose and fructose molecules, which are well-known to be reducing sugars. Glycation is described to promote the formation of covalent aggregates and to decrease the bioactivity of antibodies [150,151].

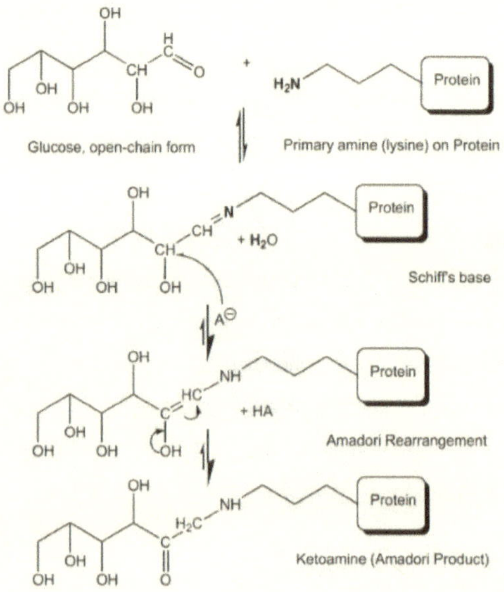

Fig. 30. Glycation reaction between glucose and the primary amine of the lysine side chain [151].

III.2.1.5 Fragmentation

The fragmentation is strongly pH dependent and it can be catalysed by metals or radicals. Covalent bonds are cleaved during fragmentation, either spontaneously or enzymatically. The cleavage of peptide bond produces low molecular weight species (LMWS). Fragmentation mainly occurs in the hinge region due to its local structural dynamic (i.e. flexibility) and accessibility [152]. Peptide bond cleavage is more prone to occur on amino acid residues such as aspartic acid, asparagine, glycine, cystein, threonine or serine.

For instance, the aspartic acid C-terminal peptide bond is one of the most frequent cleavage sites under acidic conditions. The mechanism is based on the nucleophilic attack of the ionized carboxylate (aspartic acid side chain) on the protonated carbonyl of the peptide bond chain. An N-terminal peptide with an aspartic anhydride is formed. This highly reactive intermediate may be hydrolysed to an aspartic acid residue. It has been observed that a pH value between 1 and 3 promotes such reaction, with the rate of reaction decreasing with an increase in the pH. As previously mentioned, asparagine residues can be subject to deamidation issues and form an aspartic acid residue by direct hydrolysis (low pH conditions). This residue can act as a potential site of fragmentation [153].

LMWS are detected using analytical methods such as size exclusion chromatography (SEC), mass spectrometry, sodium dodecyl sulfate-poly acrylamide gel electrophoresis and dynamic light scattering [152].

III.2.2 Physical degradation

Physical degradation may be initiated by chemical degradation of the primary structure of proteins (or peptides). The conformation of proteins evolves and adapts to the change in its environment (flexible structure). The modification of the conformation can lead to physical instabilities such as surface adsorption or aggregation. Physical instabilities usually induce a loss of functional activity and may trigger immunogenic response.

III.2.2.1 Denaturation

Denaturation corresponds to the loss of higher order structure of the protein due to an unfolding process. The higher order structure refers to the secondary, tertiary and the quaternary structures of the protein [154].

Protein denaturation refers to the unfolding of the macromolecule and the loss of its 3D structure. Various stresses can induce denaturation, such as thermal stress, mechanical stress, interfaces or chemical factors [155]. In the native form of the protein, the hydrophobic amino acid residues are buried inward to minimize their contact with water. During denaturation, these hydrophobic parts are exposed to the surrounding environment. The exposure of hydrophobic parts increases the risk of aggregation or surface adsorption. Denaturation can occur in both solid and liquid states as well as during a drying process [139,156].

III.2.2.2 Aggregation

Briefly, aggregation involves protein-protein interactions which initially generate dimers or trimers. Their growth may generate subvisible or visible particles. Species such as dimers, oligomers or multimers are usually described as high molecular weight species (HMWS). The protein-protein interactions are directly in relation with two stability concepts: conformation stability (folded-unfolded) and colloidal stability (self-association) (Fig. 31) [157].

The initial oligomerization is compared to a nucleation (i.e. growing process) which depends on the protein's conformation stability. The conformation of a protein evolves over time to adapt its structure to the vicinity. The change of conformation may expose hydrophobic residues of the protein due to an unfolding process [150]. The tertiary structure of proteins is mainly promoted by non-covalent bonds, and hydrophobic amino acids are folded inward to avoid water exposure. The non-covalency means that any changes in the physical or chemical environment may lead to denaturation [158]. Association between hydrophobic residues of the protein occurs to minimize the unfavourable contact with water. In multi-domain proteins, such as mAb, the denaturation can occur independently in different domains (F_{ab} or F_c) (Fig. 31). Several stresses, such as acidic pH, the use of organic solvents or high temperatures, may induce unfolding issues. Conformational stability influences the nucleation.

Proteins are both charged and amphiphilic macromolecules that can self-associate in clusters. Self-association is mainly driven by electrostatic interactions. Moreover, self-association is concentration-dependent and increases rapidly at high concentrations. The distance between proteins decreases at high concentrations, and monomers are more prone to associate in clusters. The nucleation rate can increase rapidly with high concentrations due to the reduced distance between proteins [150].

Aggregation is mainly irreversible due to the decrease in free energy in the formation of aggregates (i.e. thermodynamically stable state). Reversibility of aggregation is possible at the early stage of the process. Aggregation issues lead to a more stable state because of the formation of β-sheet conformations. Irreversible aggregation is described as the formation of nuclei. Nucleation and growth mechanisms are sometimes used to express the aggregation formation of proteins from the native and unfolded states towards aggregates (i.e. oligomers) and then to larger structures (Fig. 31). Irreversible aggregation is dependent on the unfolding or partial unfolding formation, which is the rate-limiting step of the process [140,157,159,160].

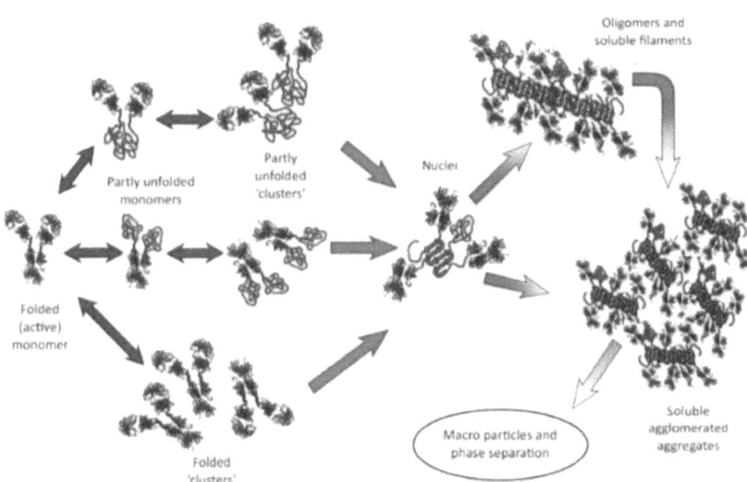

Fig. 31. mAb aggregation mechanisms. The folded clusters correspond to the self-assembly (reversible) of a native protein (oligomer). The partly unfolded monomers are separated into Fc domain denaturation, above, and the unfolding Fab domains are represented as "partly unfolded monomers". The red part on the scheme illustrates the hydrophobic patches section [157].

The basis of mAb activity is performed by its native and glomerular state (i.e. monomer). Any change in the native state tends to a loss of function and may trigger an immunogenicity response. In the case of immunogenicity, mAb is targeted by the immune system and the patient is no longer sensitive to the treatment [157]. Preservation of the integrity of the tertiary structure of the biotherapeutic is the main goal when formulating such macromolecules, to maintain their stability and therapeutic activity. Therefore the stability of a mAb during its formulation depends on the physical and chemical environment, such as temperature, pH, ionic strength, pressure and excipients [132,140].

III.3 Formulation strategies and stress factors

Instability of proteins is a major concern when formulating biotherapeutics. Stress factors occurring during production, processing or storage are mainly responsible for conformational changes. Protein stabilization is essential to promote its stability for further processing, handling or to increase its shelf life. The presence of water in the formulation is often deleterious due to its ability to promote hydrolytic processes such as deamidation, oxidation and isomerization. Therefore, the drying of the protein before its formulation, using an adapted excipient, usually increases its stability. Unfortunately, there is no universal excipient that can be used, and both qualitative and quantitative composition of the excipient often need to be adapted to each biotherapeutic [132,140].

III.3.1 Drying processes

The drying mechanism can be divided into three steps, which may appear simultaneously: (1) a transfer of energy from the drying equipment to the solvent, (2) liquid phase transformation towards the vapour phase and (3) vapour removal from the system to obtain dry product. Various techniques are described in the literature, such as freeze drying, spray drying (SD), spray freeze drying and supercritical fluid drying. The two main techniques that are commonly used in the laboratory and the pharmaceutical industry are SD and freeze drying [161].

III.3.1.1 Spray drying

Spray Drying (SD) is a commonly used process to produce biotherapeutics in solid-state dry powder. The technology is based on the atomization of the solution/dispersion through a nozzle to generate droplets (Fig. 32). Then, the droplets are nebulized in a drying chamber and put into contact with a hot dry air (or inert gas) flow. Rapid solvent evaporation occurs at the surface of the droplets. The dried particles are subsequently separated using a cyclone and directed into a collecting tube [158]. The short residence time in the drying chamber allows drying of the solution/dispersion of biotherapeutics without affecting their structure. Several process parameters may be optimized to accelerate the evaporation of the solvent. Among these are the solution concentration, the flow rate of both feeding material and hot air, the type of stabilizers and the drying temperature. Moreover, a great advantage of the SD process is its ability to harvest powder with desired size and morphology (i.e. micron-sized) using a one-step technique. This powder is helpful for further formulation processing. Spray-dried powers are commonly used for pulmonary delivery, to produce vaccine powders for intradermal delivery or in IDDS such as controlled-release microspheres [162].

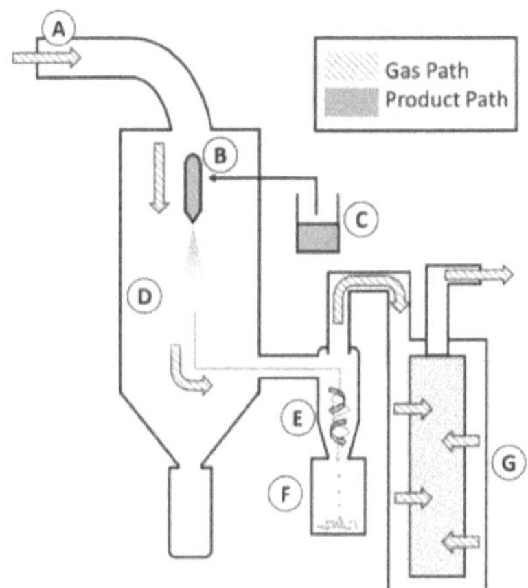

Fig. 32. SD equipment with (A) hot air flow, (B) nozzle (nebulization), (C) solution of protein, (D) drying chamber, (E) cyclone, (F) collecting tube and (G) air flow filter [163].

III.3.1.2 Freeze drying

Freeze drying, also called lyophilization, is widely described to dry biotherapeutics in solution/dispersion. The equipment is constituted of a drying chamber with controlled-temperature shelves and a condenser chamber linked through a valve [161]. The drying process starts with the freezing of the solution by decreasing the temperature of the shelves (e.g. to -40 °C). Then, primary drying acts to remove the unbounded water by a sublimation process at low pressure, keeping the product at a low temperature. Finally, unfrozen water is desorbed by increasing the product/shelf temperature to 25-50 °C [141]. The process is based on these successive steps: freezing and drying. Stabilization of protein may be performed with the addition of cryoprotectants (protection against freezing) and lyoprotectants (protection against drying). Denaturation and aggregation of proteins may be influenced by pH shifts, an increase in protein/excipient concentration, cold denaturation and water removal (drying). Freeze drying leads to the formation of a cake constituted of bulking agent (e.g. mannitol), protein and stabilizers. However, the cake needs further processing to be broken into fine particles [162]. Furthermore, the drawbacks of freeze drying are its cost and the time needed to obtain the dried product.

III.3.2 Stress factors influencing stability

This section focuses on the stress factors encountered by the protein during SD. Indeed, SD has been used as the drying technique to stabilize our biotherapeutics. The solid-state formulation was encapsulated into printable filaments to produce 3DP DDS.

III.3.2.1 Temperature

Temperature is one of the major stresses that may lead to protein instability. Indeed, heat increases the rate of protein unfolding and hence, the protein degradation. In liquid state, proteins are characterized by an equilibrium T_m, which corresponds to the temperature where 50% of the protein is unfolded. In the literature, the T_m is described to be usually ranged between 40 °C and 80 °C [140]. The aggregation rate increases above the T_m as well as with the extent of the flexibility of the protein. Moreover, reaching a higher temperature that the T_m increases the rate of deamidation and oxidation. In dry state, the T_g of the stabilizer matrix (e.g. sugars) is the thermal transition at which the mobility of the formulation increases. A higher thermal stability may be reached using a high-T_g stabilizer such as Tre (~ 120 °C). At a temperature above the T_g, the global mobility increases but denaturation is not necessarily induced [155]. For instance, SD of a solution of protein is usually performed at an inlet temperature higher than 100 °C to remove water. However, the outlet temperature is the most stressful parameter and needs to be kept as low as possible. The outlet temperature is the temperature to which the protein is exposed in the collecting tube [164]. In order to keep the outlet temperature lower than 100 °C, the inlet temperature may be decreased and the feed rate may be lowered to guarantee complete drying [162].

The ability of sugar to remain in a glassy state during the process or storage plays a crucial role in the stabilization of the protein. Sugars with high T_g are mostly used in the formulation of the protein. At temperatures higher than the T_g, sugars evolve in a rubbery state which lead to a high molecular mobility where vitrification is compromised. In addition, at a temperature above the T_g, the crystallization occurs easily and can either induce a loss of interaction or damage the protein structure through mechanical stresses. Consequently, sugars with high T_g such as disaccharides (e.g. Tre or Suc) or larger structures such as polysaccharides (e.g. dextran, Inu) are suitable when a stabilizing agent is submitted to high process temperatures [165].

III.3.2.2 Drying

Drying is associated with dehydration stress, which can lead to instabilities (e.g. conformational changes). Indeed, the stability of a biotherapeutic is increased by the presence of water through hydrogen bonds. Hydrogen bonding of water is lost during the drying step and needs to be replaced by suitable stabilizer compounds (e.g sugars) [155].

III.3.2.3 Interfaces

The formation of droplets increases the air-liquid interfaces, which usually promotes instabilities. The relative hydrophobicity of air, compared to water, may lead to unfolding and promotes agglomeration issues. Excipients with surface properties, such as surfactants (e.g. polysorbate) or amino acids (e.g. L-leucine), are commonly used to reduce the air-water interface tension. These molecules tend to diffuse to the air-liquid interface in competition with the protein to avoid its denaturation and its aggregation [163].

III.3.2.4 Residual moisture

Water is essential for the stability of the protein in liquid state as it preserves its tertiary structure. Water acts as a strong plasticizer and may induce a decrease in the T_g and thus, increases the instability of the dried formulation-loaded protein. Indeed, the decrease in the T_g increases the mobility of the whole system, which may lead to physical instability of the biotherapeutic. Moreover, as previously mentioned, numerous chemical degradations of proteins are promoted by water [155]. However, it has been previously described that a moisture percentage range between 1% and 8% (w/w) usually preserves the stability of a freeze-dried peptide [166]. A lower moisture percentage may lead to instabilities due to a critical loss of H-bonds (over-drying). The assessment of the residual moisture is carried out using thermogravimetry analysis or Karl Fisher titration [141].

III.3.3 Stabilizing agents for proteins in dry state

Several stabilizing agents can be used in liquid formulations before the drying step to prevent the degradation of proteins. The most commonly used excipients are carbohydrates, surfactants, salts, amino acids and polyols (Table 5).

Sugars are the most commonly used stabilizers for proteins which are subject to dehydration, freezing and thermal stresses. The mechanism of the sugar stabilizing effect has been described using two widely accepted physical concepts: the "water replacement theory" and the "vitrification theory" [155].

The "water replacement theory" is described as the ability of a sugar to create hydrogen bonds with the protein to promote its thermodynamic stability. During the drying process, the hydroxyl groups present in the structure of the sugar can replace the hydrogen bonds that are formed with water, maintaining the native state of the protein.

On the other hand, the "vitrification theory" is based on the formation of a rigid and amorphous glassy matrix around the protein. Protein movements are restricted and protein interaction with its environment is reduced (kinetic consideration). However, the vitrification mechanism can be more complex. Vitrification focuses on hindering global mobility (α-relaxation), but local mobility (β-relaxation) may have also a non-negligible effect. The α-relaxation represents the translation and rotational motions which are avoided with high matrix viscosity. Thus, α-relaxation is dependent on the glass transition of the matrix. The hypothesis is that physical and chemical instabilities are dependent on α-relaxation and β-relaxation, respectively [141,155,156,161,165].

Table 5. Stabilizing agents for dry state proteins and their mechanisms (adapted from [166]).

Stabilizer components	Stabilizers	Stabilization mechanism	Additional information
Amino acids	His Arginine Glycine Leucine (Leu)	Water replacement effect	- Some of them are also used as buffering agents (e.g. His, Arginine) - Leu is a hydrophobic compound with strong surface properties during drying [167].
Surfactants	Polysorbates (20 and 80) Poloxamers (188 and 407)	Protecting effect against mechanical stresses and interfacial stresses (air/liquid, solid/liquid)	- Acts as "chemical chaperone", promoting protein refolding [140].
Polyols	Sorbitol (Sor) Mannitol	Vitrification effect and/or water replacement effect	- Low T_g leading to crystallization (promoted at high concentrations or at high temperatures) [168].
Carbohydrates	Tre Suc Inulin (Inu) Dextran Cyclodextrin (e.g. 2-Hydroxypropyl-b-cylcodextrin (HPβCD)) - Glucose Maltose		- Tre – high T_g (~120 °C) - Suc – T_g ~ 60 °C - Stabilizing effect of carbohydrates is influenced by their ability to stay in an amorphous state - Polysaccharides such as Inu and Dextran: High T_g but steric hindrance and structure flexibility influence the protein-carbohydrate interactions [165]. - Reducing sugars such as glucose and maltose may induce glycation
Salts	Potassium chloride Sodium chloride Sodium sulphate Citrate	Buffering effect	

III.3.4 Strategies to sustain the duration of action of a loaded mAb

Delivery of mAb is a major challenge due to its size, stability, hydrophilicity, poor permeability through physiological membranes, susceptibility to stress factors and enzymatic degradation. Oral delivery is usually supplanted by parenteral delivery routes such as intravenous, intramuscular or subcutaneous routes. Even if these routes are invasive, they increase patient compliance and adherence to the treatment.

Biotherapeutics such as mAbs are usually administrated for chronic diseases and thus, repeated injections are needed. Consequently, mAbs are clearly good candidates to be loaded into sustained-release formulations to ensure constant therapeutic levels over time. Commonly used strategies such as micro-/nanoparticles and hydrogels have been previously reported [133,169]. All these systems have been developed to release the protein in an active form and guarantee its stability over time.

III.3.4.1 Micro-/nanoparticles

The development of polymeric microparticles for the controlled delivery of proteins or peptides has been widely investigated. PLGA derivatives are the major biodegradable polymers used in microparticle formulation. Nowadays, several peptide-loaded PLGA microparticles are marketed (e.g. Lupron Depot®, Risperdal® Consta®, Sandostatin LAR®). However, protein encapsulation using PLGA microspheres is challenging and protein stability needs to be evaluated [133].

Formulation of microparticles allows optimising some parameters such as the size distribution of the particles, their polydispersity, their porosity and their stability. The encapsulation process can be performed using SD. As PLGA derivatives are hydrophobic polymers, they require the use of volatile organic solvents to be dissolved and the avoidance of high inlet temperatures [169]. The protein may be added either in liquid (e.g. emulsion) or in a solid state (e.g. suspension). The drying step allows encapsulating proteins into the micro-/nanoparticles. Stabilizing agents need to be added to prevent protein denaturation during the process.

Microparticles are convenient DDS due their size and their ease of delivery. Practically, the microparticles are suspended in an aqueous medium and are injected using a syringe with an adapted needle [169].

III.3.4.2 Hydrogels and *in situ* gel-forming systems

These systems are based on the injection of liquid or semi-solid polymeric formulations to form a gel/solid implant *in situ*. The process includes a crosslinking between polymer chains to form a network [133]. Hydrogels swell in aqueous medium and are not dissolved in water under physiological conditions.

Several mechanisms can trigger the gel formation, such as *in situ* phase inversion or temperature-induced gel/implant formation. The former is based on an emulsion-based formulation with polymers, proteins and organic solvents. Owing to the injection *in situ* into an aqueous medium, the organic solvent leaks into water and protein compounds are encapsulated when the polymer precipitates.

Commonly used polymers are aliphatic polyesters (e.g. PLGA, PCL), and polar organic phases made of solvents such as dimethyl sulfoxide, ethanol, triacetin (TA), N-methyl pyrrolidone and glycofurol [133,169]. The latter is triggered by a change in temperature to induce sol-to-gel transformation. This process requires a thermosensitive monomer such as N-isopropylacrylamide characterized with a "low critical solution temperature" around 37 °C. The increase in temperature leads to an increase in the hydrophobic interactions in N-isopropylacrylamide backbones, which controls the collapse and form a gel.

Despite the advantages of these strategies, they are based on methods using organic solvent that is a source of instabilities for biotherapeutics. Residual solvent content needs to be fully characterized to avoid any adverse effect. Furthermore, it is difficult to regulate the burst release of these DDS due to their high porous surface. For instance, a burst release higher than 25% was reported with IgG-loaded PLGA microparticles [170]. According to the hydrogel, the homogeneity of the API and the release over time represents a limitation when DDS are developed. The formation of the hydrogel has led to high porosity and therefore to a faster drug release [171]. In this work, a monolithic DDS with a high drug loading was proposed and evaluated. The development of printable filament using HME was essential to promote the homogeneity of the system. Finally, the release of the biotherapeutic may be sustained over time with a minimal burst release.

Aims of the work

The objective of this project was to stabilize both the antibody and the system and develop a sustained-release formulation containing an antibody (i.e. mAb and Fab) using 3DP. Indeed, the novelty of the work was to investigate this technique to produce an antibody-loaded DDS with a high drug loading ($\geq$ 15% (w/w)) using the FDM technology. The use of 3DP in pharmaceutical field has increased during the last decade and the opportunity to develop IDDS seemed an attractive alternative to DDS such as microspheres. The advantages would be *(i)* to avoid the use of solvents, *(ii)* to promote a controlled release with limited burst effect, and *(iii)* to move towards personalized medicines.

To achieve this aim, the use of successive techniques was required, more precisely HME and FDM. The first challenge was to obtain an homogeneous filament made of biocompatible material with appropriate characteristics for printing. Considering that these techniques require the use of high temperatures, the second challenge was to develop a strategy to reduce these temperatures. Indeed, this is the most crucial point as the use of high temperatures would reduce the antibody stability. Finally, the third challenge was to find the best formulation of the antibody to ensure its integrity throughout the whole process.

Therefore, this work was mainly divided in four parts:

(i) The first part of this work aimed to evaluate and investigate the FDM printing parameters with the optimization of the polymeric matrix (addition of a plasticizer to a high Mw PLA). Three parameters were investigated: deposition temperature, layer thickness and deposition rate. This part was performed using placebo cylindrical and dog-bone devices. The physical and mechanical properties of the polymeric matrix were assessed.

(ii) The second part of this work consisted in the development of antibody-loaded 3DP devices using a pIgG model. This part focused on the selection of the HME and FDM parameters most adapted to building these devices. Finally, the devices were characterized in terms of content, release and pIgG stability.

(iii) Once the most suitable parameters were selected, it was interesting to investigate the feasabilty of producing mAb-loaded DDS. Therefore, this third part focused on the optimization of the mAb formulation to ensure its stability and the integrity of its structure during the process. This was done using the mAb model provided by

UCB Pharma, which was formulated using different types and ratios of stabilizers. The most promising DDS were characterized in terms of release, binding capacity, and stability over time.

(iv)   Finally, once the best process parameters were selected and the formulation optimized, it was interesting to transpose this technology to the development of a Fab-based DDS.

Experimental part

Materials and methods

I.   Materials

All the raw materials and biological entities used during this work are summarized in Table 6.

Table 6. Description of the materials used in the following experimental parts.

Products	Function	Suppliers (city, country)
Acetyl triethyl citrate	Plasticizer used to decrease the HME temperature of PLA	Sigma-Aldrich (Missouri, USA)
D-(+)-Trehalose dihydrate	Disaccharide used as stabilizer for mAb and Fab	Sigma-Aldrich (Missouri, USA)
Dichloromethane	Organic solvent used to extract protein from polymeric matrix	VWR international (Pennsylvania, USA)
Di-sodium hydrogen phosphate	Buffering agent (pH 7.0)	Merck Millipore (Massachusetts, USA)
Hydroxypropyl-β-cyclodextrin	Cyclic oligosaccharide used as a stabilizer for mAb	TCI (Tokyo, Japan)
Inulin	Polysaccharide used as a stabilizer for mAb	Alfa Aesar (Massachusetts, USA)
L-Histidine	Amino acid used as a stabilizer for mAb Buffering agent (pH 5.0 and 6.0)	Merck Millipore (Massachusetts, USA)
L-Leucine	Amino acid used as a stabilizer for mAb	Sigma-Aldrich (Missouri, USA)
Monoclonal antibody (mAb)	Biotherapeutic drug model	UCB Pharma S.A. (Braine-l'Alleud, Belgium)
Monoclonal antibody fragment (Fab)	Biotherapeutic drug model	UCB Pharma S.A. (Braine-l'Alleud, Belgium)
Polyethylene glycol 2000	Plasticizer used to decrease the HME temperature of PLGA	Merck Millipore (Massachusetts, USA)
Polyethylene glycol 400	Plasticizer used to decrease the HME temperature of PLA	Merck Millipore (Massachusetts, USA)
Polyethylene glycol - Poly(lactic-co-glycolic acid) (50:50) (mPEG-PLGA)	Biodegradable polymer used to develop a sustained-release formulation Mw = 2 kDa-20 kDa viscosity = 0.2 dL/g	Foliaplast Biological Technology Co. Ltd (Changchun, China)

Poly(lactic acid) Ingeo biopolymer 2003D (PLA Ingeo 2003D)	Biodegradable polymer used to develop a sustained-release formulation 96% L-lactide, Mw = 120 kDa ρ = 1.24 g/cm3, MFI = 6 g/10min	NatureWorks LLC (Minnetonka, USA)
Poly(lactic-co-glycolic acid) PLGA 50:50 Resomer® (RG502)	Biodegradable polymer used to develop a sustained-release formulation Mw = 7-17 kDa viscosity = 0.16-0.24 dL/g Degradation time < 3 months	Evonik Industries (Essen, Germany)
Poly(lactic-co-glycolic acid) PLGA 50:50 Purasorb® (PDLG 5004)	Biodegradable polymer used to develop a sustained-release formulation Mw = 44 kDa viscosity = 0.4 dL/g Degradation time: 1-2 months	Corbion Purac (Amsterdam, The Netherlands)
Polyclonal bovine IgG (pIgG)	Biotherapeutic drug model	Equitech-Bio Inc. (Kerrville, USA)
Polysorbate 80	Surfactant used to improve the extraction of antibodies from polymeric matrix	Sigma-Aldrich (Missouri, USA)
Sodium dihydrogen phosphate monohydrate	Buffering agent (pH 7.0)	Merck Millipore (Massachusetts, USA)
Sodium hydroxide	0.1N NaOH solution used to dissolve polymer and protein (BCA assay)	VWR international (Pennsylvania, USA)
Sorbitol	Polyol used as a stabilizer for mAb	Sigma-Aldrich (Missouri, USA)
Sucrose	Disaccharide used as a stabilizer for mAb and Fab	Sigma-Aldrich (Missouri, USA)
Triacetin	Plasticizer used to decrease the HME temperature of PLA	Sigma-Aldrich (Missouri, USA)
Triethyl acetate	Plasticizer used to decrease the HME temperature of PLA	Alfa Aesar (Massachusetts, USA)

II.   Methods

II.1 Preparation of antibody dry powder

II.1.1 Preparation of antibody feed solutions

a. Polyclonal bovine IgG (experimetal part II)

The solution of pIgG (50 mg/mL) to be spray-dried was prepared by dissolving an appropriate amount of freeze-dried powder in aqueous buffered solution (pH 6.0) made of 0.2% (w/v) His 2.1% (w/v) Tre (adapted from [172]).

b. Monoclonal antibody (experimetal part III)

The solutions of mAb to be spray-dried were made from the initial aqueous stock solution containing 160 mg/mL of mAb, 30 mM His, 200 mM Sor and 60 mM NaCl (pH 5.6). The mAb formulations were prepared by buffer exchange (BE) using a single Vivaflow® 200 cross flow cassette (Sartorius, Germany) equipped with a 30 kDa polyethersulfone membrane, coupled with a Masterflex L/S peristaltic pump (Cole-Parmer, USA). The solvent exchange was performed using a 5:1 ratio (% (v/v)) compared to the initial volume of mAb in solution. The final solution was filtered on 0.22 µm membrane using a Stericup® filtration system (Merck KGaA, Germany).

c. Monoclonal antibody fragment (experimetal part IV)

The solutions of Fab to be spray dried were made from the initial aqueous stock solution containing 50 mg/mL of Fab. The Fab formulations were prepared by BE using a single Vivaflow® 200 cross flow cassette (Sartorius, Germany) equipped with a 10 kDa polyethersulfone membrane, coupled with a Masterflex L/S peristaltic pump (Cole-Parmer, USA). The solvent exchange was performed using a 5:1 ratio (% (v/v)), compared to the initial volume of mAb in solution. The final solution was filtered on 0.22 µm membrane using a Stericup® filtration system (Merck KGaA, Germany).

II.1.2 Spray-drying process

a. SD – pIgG (experimetal part II)

The pIgG-containing solutions were spray-dried using a lab-scale Spray-Dryer B-290 (Büchi Labertechnik, Flawil, Switzerland) equipped with a 0.7 mm nozzle. The inlet air temperature was set at 130 °C; the drying air rate at 30 m³/h; the gas spray flow at 800 L/h and the solution feed rate at 3 mL/min. The outlet temperature was ranged between 75 and 80 °C (adapted from [170])

b. SD – mAb and Fab (experimetal parts III and IV)

The mAb-containing solutions were spray-dried using a lab-scale Spray-Dryer B-290 (Büchi Labertechnik, Flawil, Switzerland) equipped with a 0.7 mm nozzle. The inlet air temperature was set at 120 °C; the drying air rate at 35 m^3/h; the gas spray flow at 800 L/h and the solution feed rate at 3 mL/min (Adapted from [173]). The outlet temperature was ranged between 55 and 62 °C. The solutions were prepared in a 15 mM histidine buffer at pH 5.6. An overview of the mAb or Fab solution compositions, concentrations and mAb:excipient ratios are reported in Table 17 and Table 23 respectively. All powders were sealed in a polypropylene container and stored in a desiccator under vacuum.

II.2   Extrusion of printable filaments

II.2.1 Placebo printable filaments using single screw extruder

a. Plasticized polymer mixtures (experimetal part I)

The commercial PLA pellets were dried overnight in a vented oven at 60 °C. In a flask, 30 g of pellets were placed with 300 ml of dichloromethane-based solution containing plasticizers until complete dissolution (adapted from [174] solvent casting method). Plasticizers were fixed at 10% (w/w) in the dried materials mixture. Polymer-plasticizer blends were placed under a ventilated hood before being dried for three days in a ventilated oven at 60 °C. Then, the dried residues were roughly cut and ground in nitrogen to obtain rough pellets (3-5 mm) which could be easily introduced into the extruder.

b. Extrusion of the polymer-plasticizer mixtures (experimetal part I)

Plasticized polymer filaments were prepared using a single screw extruder (Noztek Touch, Noztek®, Shoreham-by-Sea, UK) (ø = 1.60 mm). For each extrusion, 15-20 g of pellets were fed into the extruder. The extrusion was performed at a specified extrusion temperature and the speed of the screw was adapted for each blend (Table 7). After production, the diameter of the filament was checked every 5 cm in length using an electronic measuring calliper. Portions that did not have a diameter in the acceptable range of 1.75 ± 0.05 mm were discarded. This was because the 3D printer was designed to process filaments with a diameter of 1.75 mm and only a small deviation of 0.05 mm could be tolerated without causing any issues. The filaments were stored in a vacuum desiccator prior to use.

Table 7. Hot melt extrusion temperature (T_{HME}), polymeric matrix glass transition temperature (T_g) and screw speed of each blend (n=3).

Sample	T_{HME} (°C)	T_g (°C)	Screw speed (rpm)
Pure PLA	180	53	20
PLA – 10% (w/w) PEG 400	135	42	30
PLA – 10% (w/w) TEC	148	34	37
PLA – 10% (w/w) ATEC	137	40	22
PLA – 10% (w/w) TA	142	40	30

II.2.2 Antibody-loaded printable filament HME (experimental parts II to IV)

Printable filaments were prepared from physical mixtures of raw PLGA RG502, PEG 2 kDa and antibody-containing spray-dried powders which were previously blended together using a Turbula® mixer (Willy A. Bachofen AG, Muttenz, Switzerland) (67 rpm, 30 min). The blends were manually fed into a 11-mm twin screw extruder (Process-11, Thermo Fischer Scientific, Massachusetts, USA), equipped with modular screws (length-to-diameter (L/D)-ratio 40:1), and a round die with a diameter of 1.6 mm. The barrel was heated using a gradient of temperature controlled by eight thermocouples. The feeding zone was maintained at room temperature using a water circulator. The three first segments were set at 20, 40 and 80 °C, respectively. The middle segments, from the 4th to 6th thermocouple, were set at 90 °C. The last thermocouple, which was located immediately before the die, was set at 85 °C and the die itself was set at 75 °C. For all experiments, the screw speed was set at 40 rpm during the feeding and 60 rpm when the filament was manually coiled.

II.3   3D printing of devices using fused deposition modelling

II.3.1   3D printing of placebo devices (experimental part I)

123D Design® (Autodesk®, California, USA) was used as the CAD software to design two models of devices – cylinders and dog bones – and to export them in .stl files. The specimen geometry followed the specifications outlined by the American Society for Testing and Material in the ASTM D638-14 standard for type IV tensile specimens [175–177]. The dog bone shape is the commonly used specimen for mechanical testing of material. The cylindrical devices were designed with a diameter of 4 mm and a height of 40 mm. The dog-bone devices were characterized by an overall length of 115 mm, an overall width of 19 mm and a thickness of 4 mm (Fig. 33).

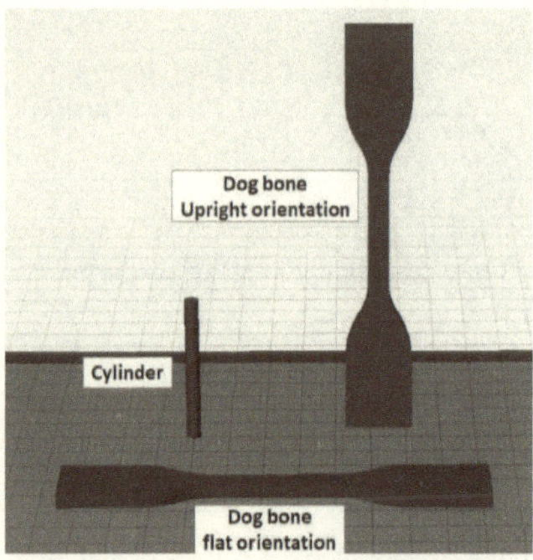

Fig. 33. Build orientations and shapes of the selected devices: a. 4 mm x 40 mm cylinder (diameter, height), b. 115 mm x 19 mm x 4 mm dog bones (overall length, overall width and thickness).

FDM was performed by a MakerBot® Replicator 2 equipped with a 0.4 mm nozzle (MakerBot® Industries, NY, USA) (Fig. 34). The MakerBot® Replicator 2 required filament with a diameter of 1.75 mm and can work with three different layer thicknesses within a range of 0.1 to 0.3 mm. The MakerBot® MarkerWare software (MakerBot® Industries, NY, USA) allows all parameters to be set, such as the deposition temperature, layer thickness and deposition rate. All the printed devices were produced using a raft of 4.0 mm (raft margin) to stabilize the structure during the printing. The raft built at the beginning of the process is a small horizontal lattice of melt filament laid down between the build platform and the device. The raft of each structure was built using the minimal print rate available in the printer parameters, 1 mm/s, without a fan and with a minimum layer duration set at 15 seconds.

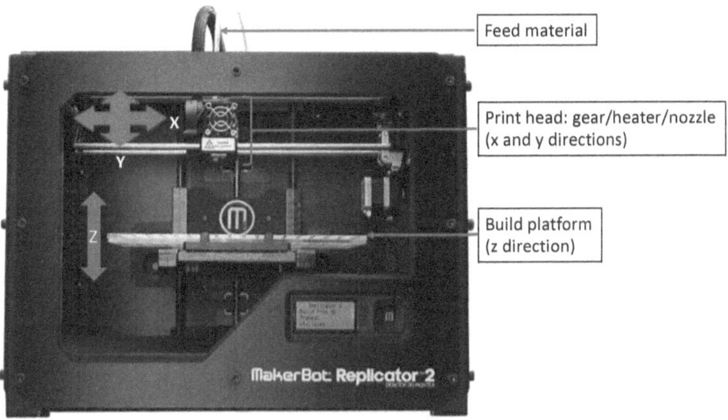

Fig. 34. Schematic image of MakerBot Replicator 2 system (feed material (filament), print head and build platform identified).

II.3.2 3D printing of pIgG-loaded devices (experimental part II)

3D CAD software ThinkerCAD™ (AutoDesk® Inc., USA) was used to design torus (Fig. 48) and cylinder devices (Fig. 54). Their dimensions were selected according to the needs of material in performing analytical tests such as the quantification of total protein assay, and extraction and dissolution tests after printing. Considering the necessity to minimize the dimensions to avoid waste of material as it was necessary to make devices for several tests (i.e. DSC, TGA, dissolution tests, extraction and BCA), the surface-area-to-volume ratio (SA/V ratio) was set at 1.67 mm^{-1} for the printed cylinder devices.

FDM was performed by a MakerBot® Replicator 2 equipped with a 0.4 mm nozzle (MakerBot® Industries, NY, USA) (Fig. 34). The deposition temperature was evaluated from 113 ± 2 °C for PEG-PLGA and RG502 and 135 °C PDLG 5004. The lowest deposition temperature was set as the minimal temperature allowing adhesion to the build platform. Printing of protein-loaded devices was performed using a layer thickness of 0.1 mm and 0.3 mm to evaluate the influence of the thickness on the potential degradation of the loaded antibody and on the antibody release profile. Furthermore, different infill percentages (50% and 100% (v/v)) were used to evaluate the influence of the device microarchitecture on the dissolution profiles of the loaded antibody.

II.3.3 3D printing of mAb- or Fab-loaded devices (experimental parts III and IV)

The design of the devices was drawn using ThinkerCAD™ and exported in .stl files (Fig. 35a). Then, the .stl file was imported into the open-source Slic3r 1.3.0. software for slicing and it was converted to a .gcode file. The dimensions of the devices were 20 x 5 x 2 mm (length, width, height) for a volume of 178.43 mm^3 (Fig. 35b).

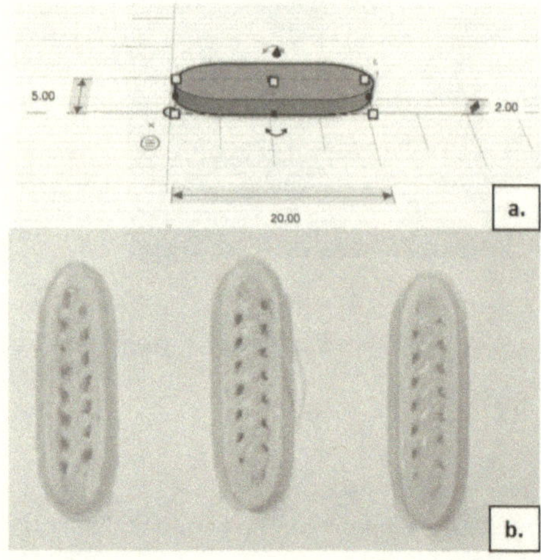

Fig. 35. a. Implantable device (20 x 5 x 2 mm (L x W x H)) designed with TinkerCad™ (AutoDesk, Inc., USA). b. 3D printed devices (100% (w/w)) obtained using the Hyrel® 30 M system.

A Hyrel® 3D system 30M printer (GA, USA), equipped with a 0.5 mm MK2-250 hot extruder, was used to print the mAb-loaded devices (Fig. 36). The temperature of the build platform did not need to be controlled. The main advantage of the printer is the ability to change the print head. The Hyrel system includes an interchangeable system with plug-and-play modular heads, which was not available with the MakerBot replicator 2 system. In this work, the MK2-250 hot extruder allowed the printing of devices using mAb- (or Fab)-loaded filament as the starting material. Indeed, this modular head reduced the traction from the gear and maintained the filament shape by using the integrated cooling fan. Consequently, nozzle clogging and squeezing of the filament were avoided.

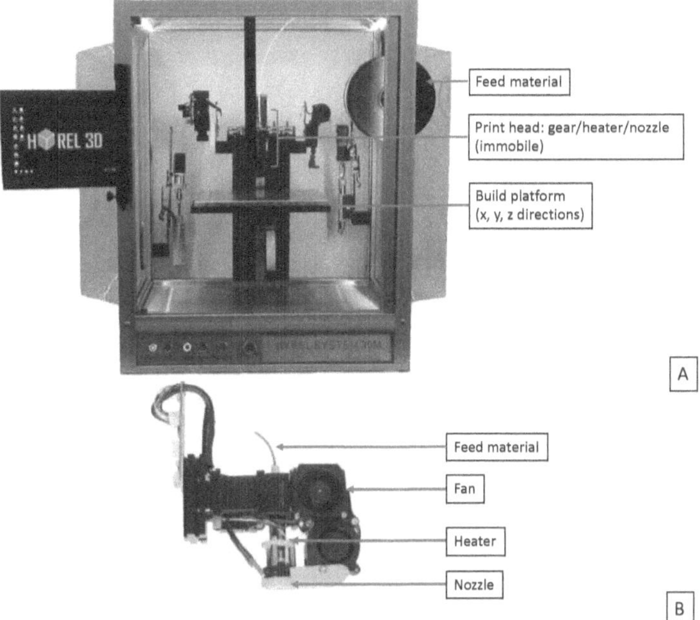

Fig. 36. Schematic image of a fused deposition modelling (FDM) system: (A) Hyrel System 30M (feed material, immobile print head, moving build platform (x, y, z directions)) and (B) MK2-250 modular head designed for flexible filament (feed material, fan, heater and nozzle).

The printing temperature was set at 105 ± 2 °C. The printing speed was set at 1 mm/s for the first layer and 10 mm/s for the subsequent layers. The layer thickness of the devices was set at 0.1 mm and 0.3 mm to evaluate the influence of layer thickness on the potential degradation of the loaded mAb as well as on the mAb release profile. The printing of devices was performed with an infill density of 100% (v/v).

II.4 Analytical methods

II.4.1 Antibody characterization

II.4.1.1 UV-VIS spectrophotometry

Characterization using UV-VIS spectrophotometry was performed using the following method on both pIgG and mAb compounds. Thus, compounds are referred to using the term "protein".

a. Protein concentration (experimental parts II to IV)

The concentration of the antibody in solution was evaluated using a spectrophotometer (Cary 60 UV-Vis, Agilent, USA), equipped with a SoloVPE system (C Technologies Inc, USA) or using a SpectraMax M5 microplate reader (Molecular Devices, California, USA) at 280 nm. The concentrations were calculated using established mass attenuation coefficients (μ(pIgG):1.14 mL/mg.cm, μ(mAb): 1.33 mL/mg.cm and μ(Fab): 1.71 mL/mg.cm) or using a calibration curve plotted as the absorbance value versus known antibody concentrations.

b. Total protein assay using bicinchoninic acid colorimetric assay (experimental parts II to IV)

The amount of protein encapsulated into the PLGA matrix was determined using colorimetric detection by bicinchoninic acid (BCA) protein assay [178]. Briefly, 3DP devices (or printable filaments) of approximatively 20 mg (or 200 mg) were dissolved in 5 mL (or 50 mL) of sodium hydroxide solution (0.1 M, pH 12.8) for 5 hours and stirred at 300 rpm, at room temperature. The solutions were filtered on 0,45 µm polyvinylidene fluoride Acrodisc® syringe filters (Pall, Saint-Germain-en-Laye, France). Then, the Pierce™ "microplate procedure" was carried out to determine the amount of melt-encapsulated mAb (working range 20-2000 µg/mL). The quantification of standards and samples was performed at 562 nm on a SpectraMax M5 microplate reader (Molecular Devices, California, USA) at room temperature. Overall, the protein loading was determined as follows (Eq.1):

$$protein\ loading\ (\%) = \frac{\text{amount of melt} - \text{encapsulated protein}}{\text{amount of 3DP device}} * 100$$

Equation 1. protein loading (%) after melt-encapsulation.

II.4.1.2 Enzyme-linked immunosorbent assay (experimental parts III and IV)

The binding capacity of the mAb was assessed using an ELISA test that was developed for the targeted mAb. The data were expressed as a percentage of the sample concentration spectrophotometrically determined at 280 nm.

Briefly, a 96-well plate was coated overnight at room temperature with a goat anti-human target antibody. Then, the plate was blocked using a solution containing bovine serum albumin to reduce the non-specific binding. The compound targeted by the goat anti-human target antibody was added to the medium. The samples containing mAb were added to the 96-well plate. The bound mAb was detected using horseradish peroxidase (HRP)-conjugated goat IgG fraction to human kappa light chain (MP Biomedicals, USA), and the reaction was visualized after the addition of the chromogenic TMB substrate (Bio-Rad, USA). The colour development was stopped after 15 minutes with 0.5 N sulfuric acid. The absorbance values, which were proportional to the amount of protein in the medium, were measured at 450 nm and with 655 nm background compensation on a Spectramax M5 microplate reader (Molecular Devices, California, USA). All incubation steps were performed at room temperature and the plates were continuously shaken.

II.4.1.3 Size-exclusion chromatography

The integrity of antibody monomer as well as the evaluation of both HMWS and LMWS contents was carried out by size exclusion high performance liquid chromatography. This analysis was conducted on samples obtained either from dissolution studies or after extraction from the devices.

a. SEC – pIgG (experimental part II)

The quantification of pIgG monomers and the evaluation of both HMWS and LMWS levels were carried out using an Agilent 1100 series LC system equipped with a UV detector (Agilent Technologies, Waldbronn, Germany). A TSK Gel G3000 SWXL column (Tosoh Bioscience GmbH, Stuttgart, Germany), 7.8 mm ID x 30.0 cm in length, was used with a flow rate set at 0.5 mL/min, a volume of injection at 15 µL, and a wavelength at 280 nm. The mobile phase was a 0.2 M phosphate buffer solution (PBS), at pH 7.0. The stability of the pIgG was evaluated using the percentage of monomer loss, which corresponded to the difference in the percentage of monomers before and after the HME and 3DP processes. The molecular weight of detected species was evaluated using the Bio-Rad Gel filtration standard, a lyophilized mixture of molecular weight markers ranging from 1 350 to 670 000 Da (Bio-Rad, California, USA). SEC data were expressed as the relative level (%) of monomer, HMWS and LMWS.

b. SEC – mAb (experimental part III)

The analysis was conducted on samples obtained either from dissolution studies or after extraction from the devices. These quantifications were performed on an Agilent 1200 series

LC system equipped with a UV detector (Agilent Technologies, Waldbronn, Germany). A TSK Gel G3000 SWXL column, 7.8 mm ID x 30.0 cm in length (Tosoh Bioscience GmbH, Stuttgart, Germany), with a TSK Gel BioAssist SWXL 6.0 mm x 4.0 cm guard column (Tosoh Bioscience GmbH, Stuttgart, Germany) was used with a flow rate set at 1.0 mL/min, a volume of injection at 50 µL, and a wavelength at 280 nm. The mobile phase was PBS 0.2 M, at pH 7.0.

The stability of the mAb was evaluated using the percentage of monomer loss, which corresponded to the difference in the percentage of monomers before and after the HME and 3DP processes. SEC data were expressed as the relative level (%) of monomer, HMWS and LMWS.

c. SEC – Fab (experimental part IV)

The analysis was conducted on samples obtained either from dissolution studies or after extraction from the devices. These quantifications were performed on a Waters Acquity UPLC system equipped with a UV detector (Massachusetts, USA). A Waters Acquity UPLC BEH200 SEC column 1.7 µm, 4.6 x 300 mm (Massachusetts, USA), with a Waters Acquity UPLC BEH 200 SEC 1.7 µm, 4.6 x 30 mm guard column (Massachusetts, USA), was used with a flow rate set at 0.3 mL/min, a volume of injection at 5 µL, and a wavelength at 280 nm. The mobile phase was PBS 0.1 M, NaCl 0.1 M, at pH 7.0.

The stability of the mAb was evaluated using the percentage of monomer loss, which corresponded to the difference in the percentage of monomers before and after the HME and 3DP processes. SEC data were expressed as the relative level (%) of monomer, HMWS and LMWS.

II.4.1.4 Protein extraction from the polymeric matrix (experimental parts II to IV)

To evaluate the stability of the protein that was melt-encapsulated in both printable filaments and 3D-printed devices, samples of approximatively 10 mg were placed in a Nanosep® with 0.2 µm Bio-Inert centrifugal devices (Pall, New-York, USA) and dissolved in 0.5 mL of dichloromethane. The Nanosep® devices were stirred at 600 rpm for 2h at room temperature to dissolve the PLGA, using a Thermomixer comfort® tubes mixer (Eppendorf AG, Hamburg, Germany). The samples were centrifuged at 12 000 rpm for 10 min and the medium was withdrawn. Then, 0.5 mL of dichloromethane were added again. The samples were stirred for

5 minutes and centrifuged as previously mentioned. This step was repeated twice. Dichloromethane was removed and the Nanosep® devices containing the protein precipitate were placed for 1 hour under vacuum to remove potential residual solvent. Then, 0.5 mL of PBS (0.2 M, pH 7.0), containing 0.02% w/w of polysorbate 80, were added in the tube to solubilize the protein before being stirred at 600 rpm for 2 hours. The Nanosep® devices were centrifuged 10 min at 12 000 rpm (Adapted from [172]). The protein stability was evaluated by SEC.

II.4.2 Dissolution test (experimental parts II to IV)

To evaluate the dissolution profile of the loaded protein from 3DP DDS, *in vitro* dissolution studies were performed. 3DP devices were placed in 2 mL Eppendorf® tubes filled with 1 mL of PBS (0.2 M, pH 7.0, 37 °C) and stirred at 600 rpm using a Thermomixer comfort® tubes mixer (Eppendorf AG, Hamburg, Germany) (adapted from [170]). At predetermined times, 1 mL of medium was withdrawn, collected and filtrated on 0.45 µm PVDF Acrodisc® syringe filters (Pall, Saint-Germain-en-Laye, France). A similar volume of fresh buffer replaced the withdrawn medium. The filtrated solutions were analysed using SEC equipment with a UV detector at 280 nm.

At each sampling time point, the potential pH modification of the dissolution medium was evaluated using a pH-meter (Mettler-Toledo, USA). Measurements were carried out at room temperature (n=3).

II.5 Polymer, filament and device characterizations

II.5.1 Thermomechanical properties

II.5.1.1 Differential scanning calorimetry (experimental parts I to IV)

DSC analyses were performed on a Q2000 heat flux differential scanning calorimeter (TA Instruments, Delaware, USA) equipped with a cooling system. Nitrogen gas was used as purge gas (flow rate = 50 mL/min) and data were collected with TA Instruments Universal Analysis 2000® software. Samples of 5-10 mg were introduced into TA Instruments aluminium pans and sealed at time zero with a lid made of the same material to evaluate the thermal properties (i.e. the T_g, determined at the midpoint of the transitions; the cold crystallization temperature (T_c); and the T_m, determined as the midpoint temperature of the endotherms) of the filaments. The reference specimen consisted of an empty sealed pan.

a. PLA-based materials (experimental part I)

During the first cycle, the oven was heated from -20 °C to 200 °C at 10 °C/min. During the second cycle, the samples were cooled to -20 °C before being heated again to 200 °C at 10 °C/min. Tg, Tc and Tm were evaluated during the second heating cycle. The degree of crystallinity (χc) was calculated using the following equation (Equation 2)[179]:

$$\chi_c = \frac{\Delta H_m - \Delta H_c}{\Delta H \frac{0}{m}} \times 100$$

Equation 2. Degree of crystallinity calculation.

where ΔH_m is the melting enthalpy, ΔH_c is the enthalpy of cold crystallization achieved during the first heating cycle and ΔH 0/m is the melting enthalpy of PLA 100% crystalline (93 J/g) [180]. All the results were calculated using the PLA quantity after subtraction of the 10% (w/w) of plasticizer.

b. PLGA-based material (experimental parts II to IV)

During the first cycle, the oven was heated up from -50 °C to 150 °C at 10 °C/min. During the second cycle, the samples were cooled to -50 °C before being heated again to 150 °C at 10 °C/min.

II.5.1.2 Thermogravimetric analysis (experimental parts I to IV)

TGA was used to measure both the residual solvent, the residual moisture contents and the thermal stability of materials. TGA was performed on a Q500 thermogravimetric analyzer (TA Instruments, Delaware, USA), equipped with a balance with a sensitivity of 0.1 µg. Nitrogen was used as the purge gas (flow rate = 60 mL/min.). Samples of 5-8 mg were loaded into platinum pans to assess the thermal stability of both plasticizers and polymers. The samples were heated at 10 °C/min from 30 °C to 600 °C. Data collection and analysis were performed using TA Instruments® Trios 4.5.0 software.

II.5.1.3 Mechanical properties (experimental part I)

The tensile testing was carried out using a Lloyd LR 10K (Ametek Inc., Pennsylvania, USA) with a load capacity of 10 kN. The 3D-printed dog-bone specimens used for tensile tests were in accordance with ASTM D638 (type IV). The reported values were the average of at least three measurements. The testing speed was set at 10 mm/min. Young's modulus, elongation at break and tensile strength were obtained using NEXYGEN™ software (Ametek Inc, Pennsylvania, USA).

II.5.1.4 Melt flow index (experimental part I)

A Davenport MFI-10 (Ametek Inc., Pennsylvania, USA) melt-flow indexer was used to evaluate the flowability of the melt. Material was cut into small pieces of around 5 mm before analysis. The ASTM standard test D1238 was used at 190 °C and a 2.16 kg load (ASTM D1238, 2013). Melt-flow index (MFI) analyses were performed to evaluate the plasticizer effect on the PLA Ingeo 2003D viscosity and to correlate the amount of matter extruded during the printing process. The evaluation of the MFI was performed using two other temperatures following the design of experiment (DoE) (173 and 155 °C) with a standard weight of a 2.16 kg load.

II.5.2 Gel permeation chromatography (experimental part III)

The decrease in polymer Mw of PLGA during the drug release was assessed using gel permeation chromatography (GPC). The protocol was similar to that used for the dissolution test. At predetermined times, devices were withdrawn and dried under vacuum for 24h. Samples of 5 mg were dissolved in chloroform. GPC analysis was performed on an Agilent liquid chromatograph (Agilent Technologies®, USA) equipped with an Agilent DRI refractive index detector and three columns: a PL gel 5 mm guard column (Polymer Laboratories®, Ltd, UK) and two PL gel mixed-B 5μm columns (columns for separation of polystyrene with a Mw ranging from 200 to 4 x 10^5 g/mol). Chloroform was used as the mobile phase at a flow rate of 1 mL/min at 30 °C. Molecular weights were calculated using polystyrene standards.

II.6 Morphological analysis (experimental part I and II)

The surface of the printed cylinder devices was visualized by scanning electron microscopy (SEM) using a JSM-600 scanning electron microscope (Jeol, Tokyo, Japan). Devices were fixed onto a carbon tape and coated with gold for 3 x 90 s at 40 mA using a Balzers SCD 030 (Balzers Union Ltd., Liechtenstein) under argon atmosphere at 10 mbar.

II.7 Statistical analysis

II.7.1 Experimental design (experimental part I)

FDM was performed by a MakerBot® Replicator 2 equipped with a 0.4 mm nozzle (MakerBot® Industries, New-York, USA). To investigate the mechanical properties (i.e. tensile strength,

Young's modulus, elongation at break) of the printed dog bones and the weight of the cylindrical devices, an experimental design was performed. Cylinders were characterized in terms of weight (Research RC 210 P MC1 0.01 mg analytical balance; Sartorius, Göttingen, Germany; n = 3). The dog-bone devices were printed in an upright orientation to evaluate the adhesion between the layers and followed the flat direction to evaluate the effect of the plasticizers on the mechanical properties. The design provided a fact-based approach, highlighting the printer performances, the relationship between variables and the influences of variables on a selected response. For these reasons, it was decided to perform first a screening design to evaluate the principal effects of parameters before optimization. The design was created using JMP statistical software (SAS Institute Inc., North Carolina, USA). The factors and levels considered in the design for the 3DP process are shown in Table 8: the deposition temperatures of the printing process, which were within the range 155 °C to 190 °C; the layer thickness of the strand during the printing process, to evaluate its influence on the layer adherence and on the device morphology; the deposition rate of the melt polymer on the build platform; and the influence of the plasticizer on the thermomechanical properties of the polymer and during the printing process. The impact of the evaluated factors was analysed using the least square regression method. An ANOVA was used to validate the statistical model.

Table 8. Factors and levels applied in the experimental design.

Factors	Levels
Deposition temperature (°C)	155, 173, 190
Layer thickness (mm)	0.1, 0.2, 0.3
Deposition rate (mm/s)	1, 88, 175
Plasticizers	ATEC, PEG 400, TEC, TA

II.7.2 Similarity factor data analysis (experimental parts II, III and IV)

The release profiles from 3DP devices were compared by calculating and comparing the similarity factor (f_2) according to the European Medicines Agency (EMA) guidance [181]. The f_2 is a logarithmic transformation of the sum-squared error of differences between the test and reference products over all time points, n *(Eq 3)*

$$f_2 = 50 \log\{[1 + \frac{1}{n} \sum_{t=1}^{n} (R_t - T_t)^2]^{-0.5} \times 100\}$$

Equation 3: f_2 factor

where R_t is the percentage dissolved at each time point for the reference and T_t is the percentage dissolved at each time point for the test formulation. The similarity of release profile was suggested with a f2 value between 50 and 100 [182].

II.7.3 Data analysis (experimental parts III and IV)

All experiments were performed in triplicate, unless otherwise specified. Prism 8 software (GraphPad software, USA) was used for statistical analysis. The results are expressed as a mean ± standard deviation. Statistical significance was determined at p-value < 0.05 using ANOVA and Tukey's or Dunnett's post-hoc test (as recommended by Prism software).

Part I - Development of placebo devices using fused deposition modelling

I. Introduction

The aim of this part was to assess the feasibility of printing devices by FDM technology. However, in contrast to the existing literature in this research area, it was decided to systematically explore the effect of various parameters using a single thermoplastic polymer (PLA) combined with different commonly used plasticizers (i.e. TA, ATEC, TEC, PEG 400) at the same percentage (10 % (w/w)). Two models of devices were experimented: cylinders and dog bones. A completed DoE was set to explore as far as possible the influence of the various printing parameters on the physical properties of the devices. Printing parameters evaluated were the deposition temperature (155, 173 and 190 °C), the layer thickness (0.1, 0.2 and 0.3 mm) and the deposition rate (1, 88 and 175 mm/s).

This study was conducted on a PLA with an Mw of 120 kDa, which required a high printing temperature. Plasticizers are small Mw compounds that can be added to polymeric matrix to decrease the T_g. In the pharmaceutical field, the ability to decrease both HME and FDM temperatures is very valuable. Indeed, high temperatures may lead to the degradation of drug compounds. This optimization and characterization study was performed on placebo devices, with a view to including antibodies in the next steps of this book.

II. Results and discussion

II.1 Formula and characteristics of the filament

The neat thermoplastic polymer PLA Ingeo 2003D was blended with four different plasticizers using a solvent evaporation method to obtain a homogeneous mixture before the extrusion process. The ratio of plasticizer (10% (w/w)) was considered miscible with the PLA after evaporation, in accordance with the miscibility study of Baiardo et al. [174]. The researchers discussed the miscibility of monomeric and polymeric plasticizers into the PLA. These plasticizers were selected because of their widespread use in pharmaceutics with PLA [183,184]. The addition of plasticizers is essential to soften the polymer, to decrease its brittleness and to enhance the processability of the polymer at relatively low process temperatures [185]. Furthermore, the aim of this study was to be able to reach the lowest temperatures of both HME and FDM by adding plasticizers. TGA was performed on filaments to evaluate the residual amount of dichloromethane after extrusion. After three days in a ventilated oven at 60 °C, no weight loss was observed above the boiling temperature of the solvent (~ 40 °C) (data not shown), which meant that it was assumed to be completely removed. The complete elimination of the solvent inside the filament was shown to be essential as it was previously demonstrated that residual solvent may have a plasticizing effect [65]. From a pharmaceutical point of view, organic solvents are subject to regulation and guidelines. Organic solvents are divided into different classes (i.e. class 1, 2 and 3) according to their toxicity and the content level. For instance, dichloromethane is in class 2 and its use should be limited to avoid toxicity to the patient [186]. Moreover, residual solvent may lead to the creation of air bubbles during HME and weaken the PLA filament. To interpret properly the data from the DoE and the influence of the plasticizers on the printing process, it was necessary to verify that no interference would be generated by the presence of residual solvent. The plasticizer ratio was selected after experimental testing of different percentages (10, 20 and 30% (w/w)). With percentages higher than 10% (w/w), the diameter of the extruded filament was not in the printability range of 1.75 ± 0.05 mm. This result was probably due to the inherent limitations of the single-screw extruder (Noztek Touch, Noztek®, UK). Interestingly, it was observed that the diameter of the filament was greatly influenced by the speed of the screw. Indeed, there were swelling issues, which is also called the "Barus effect", when the screw speed increased. This phenomenon has been described in the literature and can be explained by the viscoelastic properties of polymer. When polymer goes through the die at a relatively high velocity, its chains relax. This has led to an increase in the diameter of the filament when melt emerged from the die [187]. When a ratio higher than 10% (w/w) of plasticizer was used, the cooling step became more important due to the decrease in viscosity of the extruded filament. With 10% (w/w) of plasticizer, the limitation of the filament diameter was achieved by adapting the temperature and screw speed (Table 9). All filaments were produced using an extruder manually fed with the polymer-plasticizer mixture (as described in 'Materials and methods' – section II.2.1). For each of them, the T_{HME} and screw speed were adapted to guarantee the flow of the polymeric matrix through the die. A constant flow at the die allowed a filament with the expected diameter of 1.75 mm to be obtained. After the extrusion, the filament was manually rolled around a cylindric container. The cylindric container was put in an oven at 60 °C for 5 minutes to guarantee a constant enrolled state to facilitate the storage of the filaments.

Table 9. Extrusion temperature (T_{HME}), screw speed (rpm), glass transition temperature (T_g), crystallization temperature (T_c), ΔHc, melting temperature (T_m), melting enthalpy (ΔHm) and degree of crystallinity (χ_c) for neat and plasticized PLA samples obtained using DSC measurement.

Samples	T_{HME} (°C)	Screw speeds (rpm)	T_g (°C)	T_c (°C)	ΔH_c (J/g$_{PLA}$)	T_m (°C)	ΔH_m (J/g$_{PLA}$)	(χ_c) (%)
Pure PLA	180	20	53	110	25	150	28	3
PLA-10% (w/w) ATEC	137	22	42	102	28	148	30	2
PLA-10% (w/w) PEG 400	135	30	34	97	27	148	32	5
PLA-10% (w/w) TA	142	30	40	99	27	147	29	2
PLA-10% (w/w) TEC	148	37	40	98	25	147	30	5

As expected, the T_{HME} of the pure PLA was reduced from 180 °C to 135, 148, 137 and 142 °C after blending with 10% (w/w) of PEG 400, TEC, ATEC and TA, respectively (Table 9). The lowest T_{HME} values of 135 and 137 °C were obtained with PEG 400 and ATEC, respectively. Previous work explained that the role of plasticizers is to increase the free volume and minimize the chain interactions in the polymer structure [188]. Interestingly, the PEG 400 and ATEC were the highest Mw compounds added to the PLA in this study. However, at 148 °C the decrease in the T_{HME} was lower with TEC compared to other blends. This was despite the polar interaction between the ester groups of polymer and citrate compounds, which ensured a good solubility of the blend [188].

The thermal properties of the extruded filaments were investigated by DSC (as described in 'Materials and methods' – section II.5.1.1a) (Fig. 37). The thermograms showed an endothermic transition (T_g), an exothermic peak related to the cold crystallization (T_c) and an endothermic peak (T_m) of the material. The extruded pure PLA was characterized by a T_g at 53 °C, a T_c at 110 °C and a T_m at 146 °C. As expected, the T_g of the blends shifted to lower temperatures due to the addition of the plasticizers (Table 9). The highest decrease in T_g value was obtained with the addition of PEG 400 as the T_g was lowered from 53 °C to 34 °C.

Furthermore, the addition of plasticizer in the thermoplastic polymer induced higher chain mobility and so a faster crystallization rate during the second heating cycle (Fig. 37) [189].

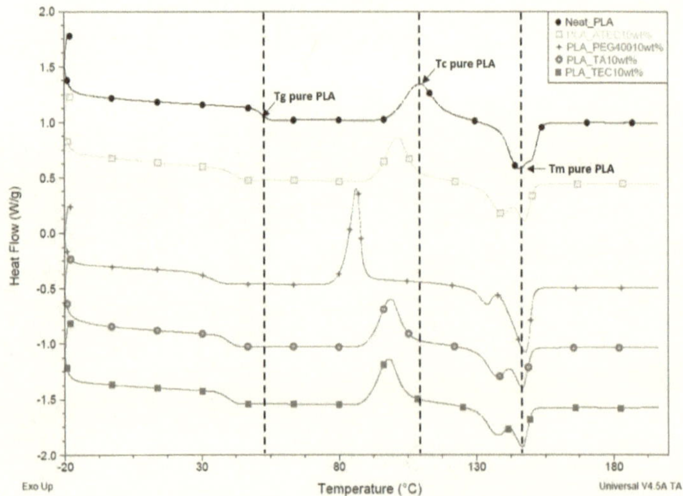

Fig. 37. Comparison of DSC thermograms of the neat PLA (●) and plasticized PLA with ATEC (◻), TA (o), TEC (■) and PEG 400 (*) captured during the second heating cycle.

However, the DSC cooling cycles showed no crystallization peak. Raw PLA and its blends are not able to crystallize at a cooling rate of 10 °C/min [190]. The χ_c may be influenced by the thermomechanical properties of the PLA (Table 9). As observed, the crystallinity of the PLA increased, from 3 to 5%, when PEG 400 and TEC were added. Chain mobility was promoted with the presence of plasticizer and explained this observation [191]. Interestingly, a lower crystallinity was observed with the addition of ATEC and TA as plasticizers (2%). As a reminder, the precision of this method is described as 0.1% in the manufacturer's specifications.

In addition, the melting peak of both raw and plasticized PLA was not defined as a single peak but as a double peak. The literature reports that these melting peaks correspond to the crystalline structure (α- and α'-forms) of the PLA and the original crystalline structure recrystallization, respectively, by lamellar rearrangement [192,193].

The DSC thermograms showed an influence from the plasticizer on the T_g and the T_{HME} of the blend (Table 9). However, the variation in T_{HME} was influenced by the plasticizer and was not only dependent on the decrease in the T_g. The T_{HME} was higher with the neat PLA and when the PLA was plasticized with 10% (w/w) of TEC. These results were related to the higher viscosity of the matter in both situations.

TGA were performed on both neat and plasticized PLA filaments (as described in 'Materials and methods' – section II.5.1.2) (Fig. 38). The thermal stability of PLA after the addition of plasticizers could be modified due to the higher mobility of the polymer chains. It was observed that the mass of the sample started to decrease at lower temperatures when plasticizers were added compared to neat PLA. The weight loss curve derivatives were analysed to assess the thermal stability of the filaments at the selected range of printing temperatures (155 to 190 °C). The derivative thermogravimetry (DTG) curves of both pure and plasticized PLA showed that degradation appeared above 200 °C (Fig. 38). However, the filament made of PLA and PEG 400 blend was less subject to degradation than those made with other plasticizers. The shift is more obvious if small molecules are added into the polymer matrix, due to their thermal stability. Furthermore, the thermal stability with the PEG 400 was higher than that from the use of the three other plasticizers (i.e. ATEC, TA, TEC). According to Li and co-workers, the shift was due to the degradation of the plasticizer when the initial temperature of degradation of the plasticizers was reached, and promoted the degradation of PLA [193].

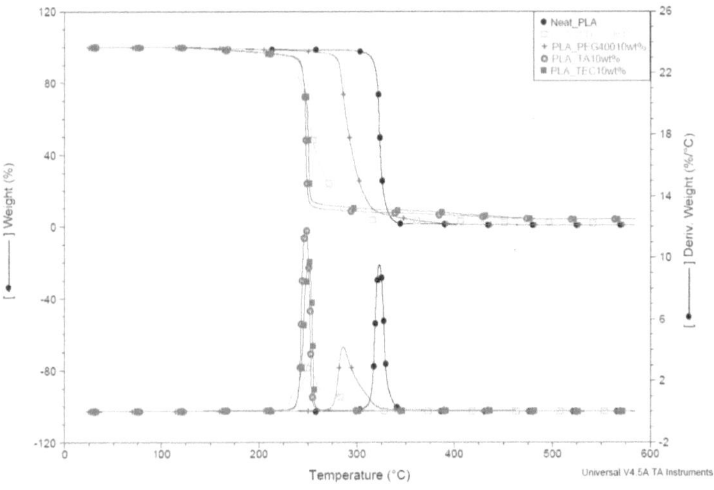

Fig. 38. Comparison of the TGA (above) and DTG (below) thermograms of the neat PLA (•) and plasticized PLA with ATEC (■), TA (o), TEC (■) and PEG 400 (*).

II.2 Melt flow index analysis of the filaments

As recommended by Fuenmayor and co-workers, MFI analysis was performed to evaluate the ability of the matter to flow through the printer nozzle at the three selected temperatures [194]. These three temperatures (i.e. 155, 173 and 190 °C) were determined by performing preliminary experiments on plasticized PLA. The lowest temperature corresponded to that at which the devices can be printed at a minimum deposition temperature adapted to all blends. The highest temperature corresponded to the temperature at which the devices can be printed before the degradation of the filament, based on TGA data. The MFI of the filaments were evaluated according to the ASTM D1238 norms (as described in 'Materials and methods' – section II.5.1.4).

At 190 °C, the MFI of the pure PLA was found to be 7.3 g/10min. At 173 °C, the MFI of raw PLA decreased even more, to 3.7 g/10min (Fig. 39). At 155 °C, PLA flowed at only 2.0 g/10min. As shown, it was clearly demonstrated that the flowability of this thermoplastic polymer was reduced when the temperature was decreased.

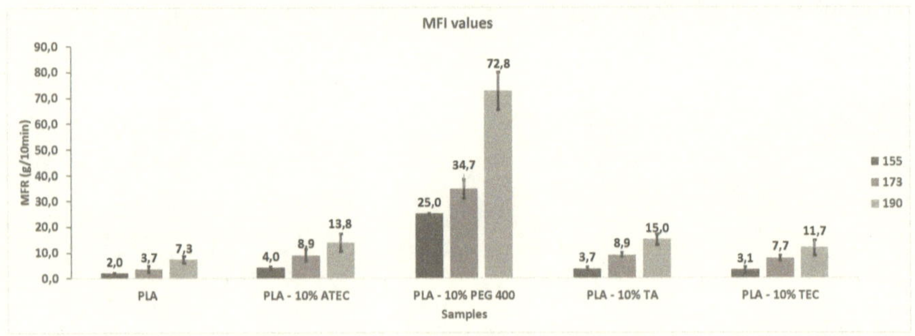

Fig. 39. MFI results (g/10min) of the neat and plasticized PLA following the selected temperatures (155 °C (blue), 173 °C (orange), 190 °C (grey) (n=3)).

The addition of 10% (w/w) of plasticizer made it possible to obtain a flow of PLA at the three temperatures tested. Regardless of the temperature, the MFI were enhanced in comparison to that of pure PLA. However, the nature of the plasticizers influenced the flowing behaviour of the polymer (Fig. 39). Indeed, it was clearly demonstrated that the addition of PEG 400 increased the MFI to a greater extent than that observed with the other plasticizers, regardless of the evaluated temperature (Fig. 39).

Recently, Wang and co-workers screened different commercial PLA and concluded that a MFI value of 10 g/10min was necessary to obtain 3D devices with an acceptable quality when printed between 190 and 220 °C [195]. Furthermore, they highlighted that during the melt deposition of the polymer, the importance of the plasticizer and the crystallinity need to be considered together, in addition to that of the MFI value [195]. During this work, several values were lower than the expected 10 g/10min. Interestingly, the addition of 10% (w/w) of plasticizer was slightly appreciable. The values of the MFI from PLA at 155 °C increased from 2.0 g/10min to 4.0, 3.7 and 3.1 g/10min with ATEC, TA and TEC respectively. In contrast, a higher MFI value (25.0 g/10 min) was observed with PEG 400. Despite the difficulty in obtaining a structure without defects, the aim of the study was to achieve results with a wide range of parameters.

II.3 Manufacture of the devices by FDM

The PLA Ingeo 2003D was printed at 230 °C using the manufacturer's specifications [196]. As the final aim of this work was to load 3D IDDS with a model of antibody, the addition of plasticizer was relevant to decrease the deposition temperature. To overcome the degradation which could take place during the printing, the influence of several plasticizers on it were evaluated. Information concerning printing protocols when plasticizers were used is missing in the literature although it could be interesting in the pharmaceutical field. In this case, the most rational approach to obtaining information about the process was to perform a DoE. The printing parameters and the influence of the plasticizer on the printing feasibility could easily be screened to identify a printing protocol which allowed the production of adequate 3DP devices.

The experimental design was established with four parameters (Table 10). Each parameter was set with a minimal and a maximal value as well as an arithmetic mean thereof. The selected DoE was established to obtain information and understand the printability of the matter using a wide range of parameters.

Table 10. Experimental design used to produce the devices.

Experiment #	Deposition temperature (°C)	Layer thickness (mm)	Deposition rate (mm/s)	Plasticizer (10% (w/w))
1	190	0.1	175	TA
2	173	0.2	88	ATEC
3	155	0.3	1	TA
4	155	0.1	175	TEC
5	190	0.1	1	ATEC
6	190	0.1	1	TA
7	155	0.3	175	ATEC
8	155	0.1	1	PEG 400
9	190	0.3	175	PEG 400
10	173	0.2	88	TEC
11	190	0.3	1	TEC
12	173	0.2	88	PEG 400

The estimation of the lowest temperature was evaluated using an empirical method. The plasticized PLA filaments were tested at several loading temperatures to identify the temperature required to promote both the loading of the filament and the adhesion of the melt onto the build platform. At 155 °C, the loading could be performed without obstruction: the plasticized thermoplastic polymer flowed properly through the nozzle of the printer and adhered to the build platform, regardless of the plasticizer used. However, to enhance the adhesion of the devices onto the platform during the printing process, blue painter's tape was systematically used (as described in 'Materials and methods' – section II.3.1) [41]. The maximal temperature was set at 190 °C to prevent the degradation of the filaments, in accordance with the DTG data (Fig. 38).

Both the deposition rate (1–175 mm/s) and the layer thickness (0.1–0.3 mm) were fixed in accordance with the manufacturer's requirements. The infill of the devices was set at 100% to evaluate the potential maximum response during the test.

During the first part of the investigation, the upright orientation was used for cylinder devices due to the high degree of shrinkage in the flat orientation (Fig. 40).

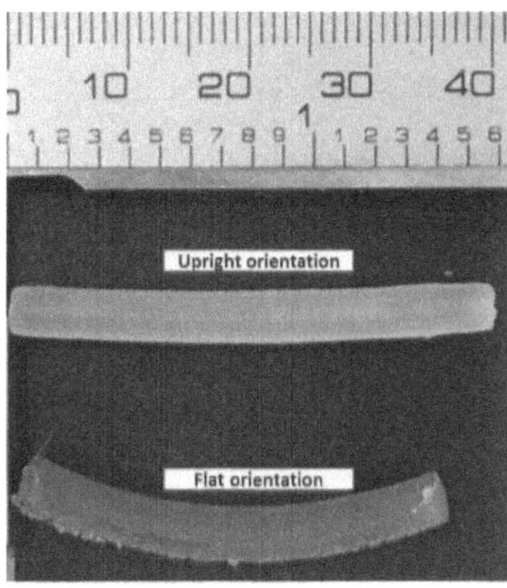

Fig. 40. Shrinkage of the cylinder device printed in the upright orientation and in the flat orientation.

The printing process was performed using a raft (small horizontal lattice of melt filament laid down between the build platform and device) to increase the adhesion of the first layer onto the build platform and to improve the stability of the devices during the whole process. The raft played a key role during the printing of the cylinders and the dog bones in the upright orientation. Indeed, due to the small area of contact between their bases (12.56 mm^2) and the build platform, both devices pitched during the printing until they were completely peeled off by the repeated back-and-forth movement of the print head. As previously described by Carneiro and co-workers, the nozzle of the 3D printer was manually adjusted at 0.36 mm to the platform and so expanded the extrusion width to enhance the overlapping of the layers of the raft [197]. Such manual adjustment of the nozzle did not interact with the printability of the devices as the build platform moved down by increments to provide the right preselected layer height.

II.4 Morphological analysis of the printed cylinder devices

SEM analysis was performed on the samples to obtain more insight into the morphology of the external surfaces of the printed devices (as described in 'Materials and methods' – section II.6) (Fig. 41). The layer height modulation at three different levels (0.1, 0.2, and 0.3 mm) could have an influence on the surface of the devices. Figure 31 shows the comparison of the external surface of samples 2, 3, 7, 8, 9 and 11, obtained from different layer heights.

As hypothesized, the increase in the height had a positive influence on the resolution of the devices. At 0.1 mm (Fig. 41a), the matter was highly embedded, probably because the build platform went down slowly and the printer nozzle, which was heated, had an extended contact area during the process, leading to the melting of the previous printed layers. The improvement of the resolution was due to the increase in the thickness to reach values of 0.2 and 0.3 mm. Interestingly, the external surface of sample 7 (Fig. 41c), which was printed at a temperature of 155 °C and at 175 mm/s, was faithful to the design, while the MFI of the initial filament (PLA-ATEC 10% (w/w)) was only 3.4 g/10min. A better resolution may be important in the future, when developing pharmaceutical IDDS, to promote a high surface area, avoid the solid-state surface obtained with 0.1 mm of layer height and promote the reproducibility of the IDDS.

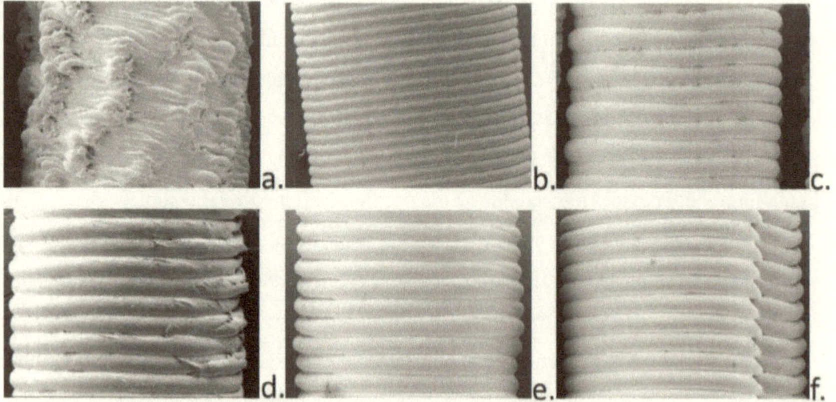

Fig. 41. SEM micrographs of the surface of cylindrical devices with : a. sample 8 (155 °C, 0.1 mm, 1 mm/s), b. sample 2 (173 °C, 0.2 mm, 88 mm/s), c. sample 7 (155 °C, 0.3 mm, 175 mm/s), d. sample 3 (155 °C, 0.3 mm, 1 mm/s), e. sample 9 (190 °C, 0.3 mm, 175 mm/s), f. sample 11 (190 °C, 0.3 mm, 1 mm/s) at 30x magnification.

II.5 Design of experiment

The DoE was performed to investigate the printability of the matter following a set of four parameters. To our knowledge, these parameters included four different plasticizers that have not already been investigated for 3DP. To visualize the effect of each parameter and the associated response, a prediction profiler was used (Fig. 42). The prediction profiler provided an overview of the responses before the discussion below, based on each effect. Furthermore, the profile can be employed to estimate the response of each experimental parameter.

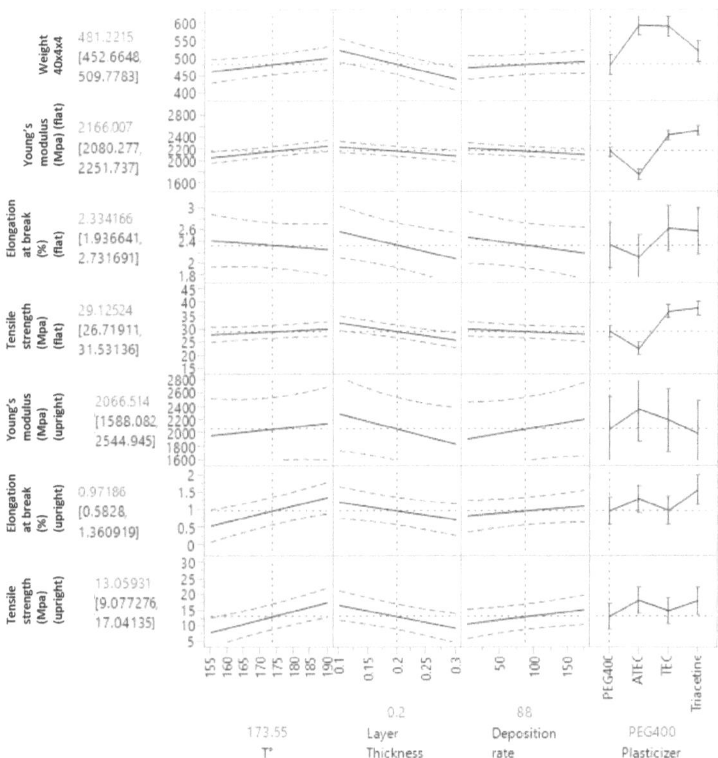

Fig. 42. Summary of the effect of the evaluated parameters (deposition temperature (T°), layer thickness (mm), deposition rate (mm/s) and type of plasticizer) on the analysed factors (weight, Young's modulus, elongation at break and tensile strength) generated during the experiments with a prediction profiler. The estimate values (y-axis, red) of those factors are according to the fixed parameters (x-axis, red). The mean value is showed using the black line and the confidence interval is represented by the blue dotted line.

113

II.5.1 The effect of the FDM process parameters on the weight of the cylinder devices

It has been demonstrated that the deposition temperature, the layer thickness and the nature of the plasticizer had a significant impact on the variability of the mass of the devices after printing (p-value < 0.05) (Fig. 42). This result may be correlated with the flow of the matter through the nozzle. The weight of the cylindrical devices increased when the deposition temperature was increased.

When the temperature rose, the flow through the nozzle increased, which was confirmed by the MFI values (Fig. 39). Higher temperatures (173 and 190 °C) allowed avoiding the clogging of the nozzle and improved the flow of the polymer melt on the platform. In contrast, an increase in the layer thickness induced a weight decrease at values higher than 0.1 mm. Chacon and co-workers explained that, when the layer thickness increased, a lower number of layers was needed to achieve the final structure [198]. Therefore, the printed devices with higher thicknesses needed less material and so were characterized by a lower weight than that expected. This observation could be attractive in adapting the loading percentage of an active molecule to a 3DP DDS. The influence of the addition of plasticizers on the weight was unexpected. Indeed, although the addition of PEG 400 to the PLA increased its MFI, it seemed that the flow of the mass was lower during the printing with this plasticizer as the weight of the device decreased.

II.5.2 The effect of the FDM parameters on the mechanical properties of the dog-bone devices

As recommended by Abdelwahab and co-workers, mechanical testing was performed on both neat and plasticized PLA dog-bone devices [199]. The brittleness of the PLA is widely known and enhancement of the mechanical properties of the material was required. The ductility of the 3DP devices was improved by the addition of plasticizers [180,185,200,201]. It was previously demonstrated that PLA was characterized by a high Young's modulus and tensile strength [174]. It was expected that the addition of plasticizers could decrease both Young's modulus and tensile strength values, with an increase in the elongation at break values. The devices were printed following the upright and the flat orientations. The flat orientation was used as typical shape to investigate the mechanical properties of the material. The adhesion between the layers was investigated on devices that were printed in the upright orientation. Furthermore, the experiments showed that the flat orientation resulted in difficulties such as shrinkage and defects in obtaining cylindrical devices. Hence, the main approach to producing devices was to print them in the upright orientation. The evaluation of the anisotropy of the mechanical response of the 3DP devices could improve the ability to print devices in the upright orientation and promote a similar structure to that initially designed. Chacon and co-workers showed that the tensile strength of a printed device could be modulated by varying only the orientation of the printing. Indeed, it was demonstrated that the tensile testing was performed parallel to the layer deposition in the case of upright samples. This observation was opposite to that observed from the flat-oriented devices. Moreover, these results were in accordance with the literature [198].

The tensile test was performed to evaluate the Young's modulus, the elongation at break and the tensile strength of the dog-bone devices.

The deposition temperature significantly modified the Young's modulus (p-value = 0.004) with the flat oriented dog bones. It was observed that an increase in the deposition temperature led to higher Young's modulus values (Fig. 43a). Indeed, considering the temperature range from 155 °C to 190 °C, the Young's modulus was able to increase from 1 556.6 ± 557.8 MPa to 2 786.4 ± 147.7 MPa for experiments 6 and 7, respectively (Table 10). For the upright orientation, the responses were significant for the elongation at break (p-value = 0.007) and for the tensile strength (p-value = 0.004) (Fig. 43a and b). The higher temperature tended to promote an increase in both mechanical properties. Indeed, the elongation at break maximum value of 2.6 ± 0.4% was observed during experiment 1 (Table 10). The tensile strength increased from 6.8 ± 2.2 MPa to 28.2 ± 1.1 MPa in the range of temperatures 155-190 °C. Torres et al. stated that when the temperature was increased, the molten state of the PLA led to a better adhesion to the previous layer [196]. The tensile strength of the upright-printed pure PLA following the manufacturer requirements at 230 °C, 90 mm/s was 19.9 ± 0.5 MPa and 47.5 ± 2.4 MPa, with a layer thickness of 0.1 and 0.3 mm, respectively. These values highlighted that the decrease in temperature succeeded in producing 3DP devices, regardless of the thickness of the layers.

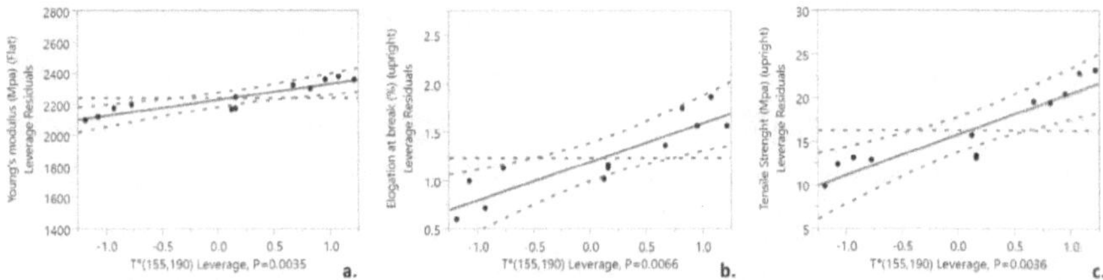

Fig. 43. Tendency of the deposition temperature for: (a) the Young's modulus in the flat orientation, (b) the elongation at break in the upright orientation, (c) the tensile strength in the upright orientation according to the experimental design given in Table 10. The mean value is represented by the red line and the confidence interval corresponds to the red dotted line.

The layer thickness significantly affected both Young's modulus (p-value = 0.01) and the tensile strength (p-value = 0.002) in the flat orientation as well as both elongation at break (p-value = 0.04) and tensile strength (p-value = 0.01) in the upright orientation (Fig. 44). Regardless of the printing orientation, an increase in the layer thickness led to lower mechanical properties. Indeed, all the mechanical properties tended to decrease when the layer thickness increased from 0.1 to 0.3 mm. The decrease in the Young's modulus values when the layer thickness increased led to a decrease in the stiffness of the device (Fig. 44a). Indeed, the stiffness of the matter has been evaluated following the Young's modulus values [198] and the decrease in both the Young's modulus and the tensile strength led to a lower stiffness of the material. Tymrak and co-workers highlighted a similar trend in their work on PLA, where a higher tensile strength was reached by lowering the layer thickness [202]. When the devices were printed in the upright orientation, the tendency was similar to that previously mentioned. A higher layer thickness tended to promote lower mechanical properties (Fig. 44c and Fig. 44d). Interestingly, Chacón and co-workers found that the upright strength increased with a higher layer thickness. Moreover, in the flat orientation, the decrease in the layer thickness increased the strength but with only a slight effect [198]. This result was different from that obtained during our experiments. In the study of Chacón et al., the effects of layer thickness, build orientation and feed rate on PLA printed devices were evaluated for the PLA mechanical properties. In the case of the present study, the deposition temperature was modulated, and plasticizers were added. However, the DoE was performed to evaluate the main effect of the selected FDM parameters.

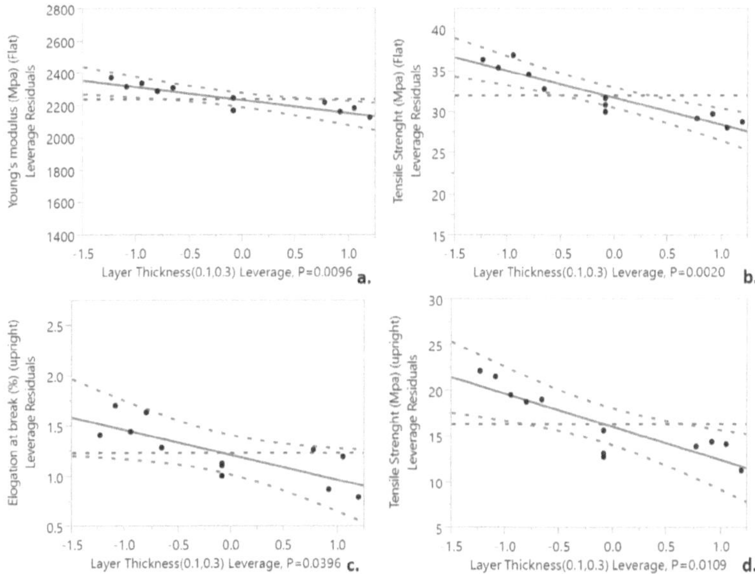

Fig. 44. Tendency of the layer thickness for: (a) Young's modulus in the flat orientation, (b) the tensile strength in the flat orientation, (c) the elongation at break in the upright orientation, (d) the tensile strength in the upright direction. The mean value is represented by the red line and the confidence interval correspond to the red dotted line.

The deposition rate was the printing parameter with the least influence on the mechanical properties (Fig. 42). Indeed, the only significant response was a slight decrease in the Young's modulus (p-value = 0.04) when the devices were printed in the flat orientation. Consequently, it may be interesting to evaluate the interaction between the deposition temperature and the deposition rate as this could explain the previous statement. A lower deposition temperature (155 °C) associated with a higher deposition rate (175 mm/s) could lead to more porous structures due to a lack of the intra-layer adhesion during the process [203].

The influence of the plasticizer on the mechanical properties was also investigated on dog bones. The significance of the results was different according to the orientation of the printing. The model responses were significant only when both Young's modulus and tensile strength values were lower than the two significant model responses. ATEC was shown to be the most significant plasticizer influencing a decrease in both Young's modulus and the tensile strength (p-value < 0.0001) (Fig. 42). The addition of ATEC to the PLA led to a sharp decrease in its stiffness and increased its ductility. In contrast, the addition of TEC and TA to the polymer matrix increased both Young's modulus and the tensile strength in the flat orientation. PEG 400 had no significant effect on the Young's modulus and had a slight effect on the tensile strength, in the same orientation. When the dog bones were printed in upright orientation, the nature of the plasticizers had a lower influence on the mechanical properties. The only significant response was obtained for the elongation at break. Moreover, TA was the only plasticizer that had a significant effect on the elongation at break. An increase in the elongation at break was observed when TA was added.

III.   Conclusion

This study showed that the addition of a plasticizer is required to decrease the processing temperatures of PLA. It was demonstrated that a higher reduction of the T_g was obtained when PEG 400 is added to the PLA. This observation demonstrated that the use of FDM may be successful for producing devices in the pharmaceutical field in further investigations to develop 3DP devices containing an antibody.

This study showed that the addition of ATEC seemed to reduce the PLA stiffness and the addition of TA promoted a better adhesion between layers. Furthermore, the stiffness of the material could also be modulated by the choice of parameters and the printing orientation. Indeed, the ductility was improved by a higher layer thickness, while a lower deposition temperature led to a less stiff material and consequently to a harmless implant for the patient. The adhesion between layers was promoted by a decrease in layer thickness and an increase in the deposition temperature. No significant effect on the deposition rate was observed with the selected DoE. The interrelationship between parameters needs to be investigated to improve knowledge about the mechanical properties of the plasticized PLA and the influence of the printing parameters.

In addition, it could be interesting to understand how the matter reacts during and after the FDM process to perform flexural testing. The orientation had a key role on the mechanical results, but the selected raster angle should be evaluated due to its ability to increase the load-bearing behaviour of the fibres deposited by the printhead. Furthermore, the addition of an active molecule into the polymer matrix will probably modify the structure as well as the thermomechanical properties.

Part II – Development of PLGA pIgG-loaded implantable devices using fused deposition modelling

I. Introduction

In the previous part, the ability to reduce the printing temperature was demonstrated by adding a plasticizer. However, despite the addition of 10% (w/w) of plasticizer, the PLA Ingeo 2003D still required a high temperature of 155 °C to be printed. This was mainly related to its high Mw of 120 kDa. As the aim of this work was the development of antibody-loaded 3DP devices and as antibodies are thermosensitive compounds, high temperatures (e.g. 155 °C) lead to their denaturation. Consequently, the use of lower Mw polymers was investigated as a strategy to reduce both HME and FDM temperatures. PLGA was selected for its biocompatibilty and its wide use in the pharmaceutical and medical fields to produce DDS. The goal of this study was to develop printable PLGA filaments and 3DP devices loaded with a pIgG as model. Both HME and 3DP were achieved to reach 20% (w/w) of loading.

PLGA derivatives are well described for the manufacturing of controlled drug release systems and represent a great potential to develop printable filaments as well as 3DP DDS. However, numerous types of PLGA derivatives are available according to their Mw and viscosity. The selection of the appropriate PLGA derivatives was essential to promote the stability as well as the sustained release of the loaded pIgG.

Printable filaments were produced using HME. Their loading and homogeneity were the mandatory parameters to ensure 3DP devices with both high loading and reproducibility. Then, the parameters of the 3DP, such as the deposition temperature, the deposition rate and fan power, were optimized.

II. Preliminary studies

This preliminary study was dedicated to the selection of a suitable polymer to perform further experiments and to develop the 3DP DDS.

The first part of this project was performed on a semi-crystalline polymer (PLA Ingeo 2003D) which required the use of relatively high temperatures (i.e. melting temperature range: 130-180 °C) to be extruded (i.e. HME and 3DP). The PLA Ingeo 2003D is inexpensive, was affordable in large amounts and is still widely described in the literature for 3DP [204,205]. However, the use of this polymer could lead to the degradation of the pIgG, with a degradation rate that was too slow to be used in IDDS.

Moreover, it is well-known that PLA is associated with local inflammation, with hydrolysis of its matrix in a smaller acidic species due to its erosion. In addition, high Mw PLA derivatives are usually preferred for use as material for tissue engineering or surgical implants [100]. Therefore, the PLGA copolymer was preferred to develop our pIgG-loaded 3DP IDDS.

II.1 Development of printable filaments using HME

II.1.1 Polymeric matrices characterizations and selection

Polymers such as PLGA are mostly used for the controlled release of small chemical entities or small macromolecules such as lysozyme, BSA and ovalbumin [128,129,206]. As the use of a relatively low temperature was essential to preserve the stability of the pIgG, the first step of this development was to select suitable PLGA derivatives (Table 11).

Two PLGA derivatives, PDLG 5004 and RG502, were characterized by different Mw of 40 kDa and 7-17 kDa and an inherent viscosity of 0.4 and 0.2 dL/g, respectively. The third was a PEG-PLGA derivative, with an Mw of 2 kDa (PEG) and 20 kDa (PLGA) and an inherent viscosity of 0.2 dL/g. The aim of this screening was to select a derivative characterized by adequate properties (i.e. Mw, viscosity) to be processed at the lowest temperature possible. Indeed, it is widely accepted that the processing temperature depends on the physicochemical properties of the polymer, such as its Mw and inherent viscosity [105,207]. Moreover, the release profile of the loaded compound and the degradation rate of the polymer also depend on its Mw.

TGA was performed to investigate the thermal stability of these polymers (Table 11). No residual moisture was observed from the raw material after being dried overnight in an oven at 37 °C (data not shown). Such information was essential as polyesters are degraded by hydrolysis, and residual moisture could increase the rate of degradation and reduce their stability during storage [122].

TGA also showed that the degradation temperature, or more precisely, the onset degradation temperature of the polymers, was around 200 °C with PDLG 5004 and PEG-PLGA while the RG502 mass loss began at 175 °C (Table 11). These values were higher than the temperatures used for both HME and 3DP. Consequently, no degradation of the polymeric matrix was expected during the manufacturing of the 3DP devices.

Table 11. Overview of the PLGA derivative and the associated glass transition temperature (T_g), the onset degradation temperature (T_{Onset}) and extrusion temperature (T_{HME}) values according to the 8 thermocouples available from feed zone to the die.

Polymer	T_g (°C)	T_{Onset} (°C)	T_{HME} (°C)
PDLG 5004	40.1 ± 0.2	200	20-40-80-100-100-100-100-100
PDLG 5004-10% (w/w) PEG 2 kDa	24.5 ± 2.7	/	20-40-80-100-100-100-100-100
PEG-PLGA	15.6 ± 0.4	200	20-40-70-80-80-80-80-82
RG502	38.0 ± 0.7	175	20-40-80-90-90-90-90-90
RG502-10% (w/w) PEG 2kDa	21.5 ± 1.2	200	20-40-80-90-90-90-85-75

DSC analyses of PLGA derivatives are summarized in Table 11. The highest T_g was observed from PDLG 5004 and RG502, with 40.1 ± 0.2 °C and 38.0 ± 0.7 °C, respectively. The PEG-PLGA copolymer was characterized by a T_g of 15.6 ± 0.4 °C. Both PDLG 5004 and RG502 were plasticized using a PEG derivative characterized by a Mw of 2 kDa.

Low Mw PEG derivatives are widely used in pharmaceutics [184]. These compounds are amphiphilic and allow a decrease in the T_g of the polymer. Indeed, their amphiphilic chains take place to the free volume of the main polymeric chains. Their plasticizing effect is mainly due to the reduction of the intrinsic interactions between the PLGA chains, which enhances their flexibility and processability. Furthermore, the addition of PEG would be interesting for the *in vitro* dissolution test as its amphiphilic properties act as a pore-former agent and allow the release of large macromolecules (i.e. biotherapeutics) [208]. PLGA erosion induces a local acidification, and the pH decrease is deleterious for the loaded compound. Pore formers, such as plasticizers, increase the degradation rate of the polymer by creating hydrophilic channels inside the DDS and then promoting the release of the loaded drug over time [130]. The addition of 10% (w/w) of PEG 2 kDa to the PLGA PDLG 5004 and RG502 using HME led to a decrease in the T_g to 24.5 ± 2.7 °C and 21.5 ± 1.2 °C, respectively (Table 11).

II.1.2 Development of printable filaments using TSE

The determination of the T_{HME} was performed on a Process 11 extruder (Thermo Fischer Scientific, Massachusetts, USA) characterized by a barrel containing double screws (Length/Diameter ratio: 40) with the basic configuration (Fig. 45b). Briefly, the extruder is divided in different parts: a feeder, a barrel containing two screws, a control panel, torque and pressure sensors and a die with a specific shape (i.e. circular, square, tubular or rectangular) (Fig. 45a). This configuration allows the matter to be well-mixed, with three mixing zones (kneading elements) which correspond to "high shear zones". Although the Process 11 is a laboratory-scale extruder, its specifications require at least 20 g of material for effective processing. The high quantity required needed to be adapted due to the high cost of raw polymer and considering the biotherapeutic compound.

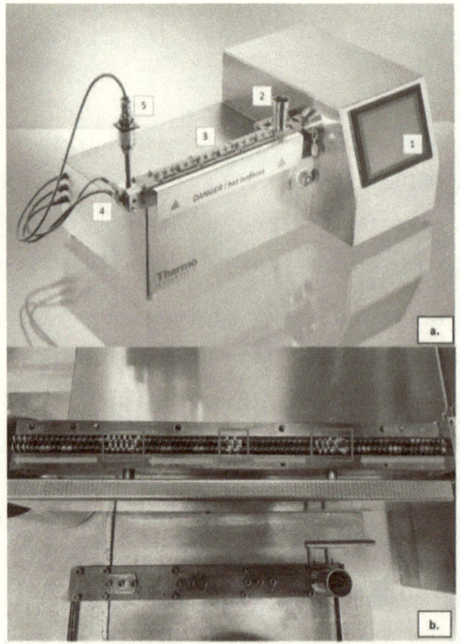

Fig. 45. **a.** Process 11 equipment with (1) the control panel; (2) the hopper; (3) the barrel containing the screws; (4) the die with temperature sensor; (5) pressure probe. **b.** The basic screw configuration with the conveying zones (green arrows) and the three kneading zones (red squares).

The use of a twin-screw extruder instead of a single screw extruder allowed to produce loaded filaments using a solvent-free process. Before the extrusion, the polymer, the plasticizer, the stabilizers and the pIgG were mixed together (as described in 'Materials and methods' – section II.2.2). As the temperature is controlled throughout the barrel to avoid over-heating due to friction, the intermeshing screws with a co-rotating movement promote the flow of the melt towards the die. Moreover, a better mixing and a higher power to homogenously disperse the active compounds into the polymeric matrix have been reported for this equipment [184].

The selection of the PLGA was done according to the temperature needed to perform the HME. Aho et al. reported that the T_{HME} is at least 10-20 °C above the T_g of selected polymer [207]. Parameters such as torque and die pressure were monitored during the process. Indeed, the torque is the strength of the motor to allow the rotation of the screws. The torque can be lowered by an increase in the temperature, which decreased the viscosity of the melt. In parallel, the die pressure is also dependent on the viscosity of the melt.

Extrusion was performed on the PDLG 5004 with an initial temperature of 50 °C at the feeding area while all the other zones were set at 70 °C and the screw speed was fixed at 40 rpm. This gradient of temperature did not allow the extrusion of filaments due to a torque higher than 100% (12 Nm). Therefore, the T_{HME} was increased to 100 °C with 40 rpm to perform extrusion and produce filaments with a diameter of 1.75 mm. The selection of this temperature provided a torque around 60% (7.2 Nm), which was adapted to extrude a filament. The first tests performed on the PDLG 5004 demonstrated that a processing temperature of at least 100 °C was necessary to avoid any interruption of the HME (Table 11). Moreover, the extrusion of the RG502 derivative was carried out at a temperature of 90 °C as reported in literature [129]. Similarly to PDLG 5004, RG502 showed a higher brittleness after HME and was unable to be further processed (i.e. by FDM).

To improve the mechanical behaviour of the filament, a plasticizer was added to PLGA derivatives. Both PDLG 5004 and RG 502 were plasticized using 10% (w/w) PEG 2 kDa.

Then, the spray dried pIgG powder (as described in 'Materials and methods' – section II.1.2a) was loaded into the polymeric matrix (i.e. PDLG 5004, RG 502 and PEG-PLGA) (Table 12). As the processing temperatures were quite high (i.e. not lower than 90 °C), the pIgG stability through thermal degradation was assessed using Tre as a stabilizer. It has been reported that stabilizers such as Tre were able to stabilize protein by water replacement or by the vitrification effect [155]. Furthermore, the high T_g (~ 120 °C) of the Tre maximizes the vitrification potential and has already been used to stabilize BSA during HME [129]. The filaments were produced with a loading of 20% (w/w).

Table 12. Theoretical compositions of printable filaments produced using HME (% (w/w)) and the temperature of each thermocouple, according to the raw polymer. Screw speed was set at 40 rpm.

HME batch number	Polymer	Polymer (% w/w)	PEG (% w/w)	Stab. (% w/w)	pIgG (% w/w)	Thermocouple temperature (°C)							
						# 1	# 2	# 3	# 4	# 5	# 6	# 7	Die
HME_1	PDLG 5004	66.8	6.7	6.3	20.2	70	100	100	100	100	100	100	100
HME_2	PEG PLGA	73.6	0.0	6.3	20.1	40	60	80	80	80	80	80	82
HME_3	RG502	66.8	6.7	6.4	20.2	40	60	90	90	90	90	83	73

*(Stab.: stabilizer (Tre))

The temperature set for HME was empirically determined using temperatures assessed with both the raw and plasticized PLGA derivatives (Table 11). As previously mentioned, the temperature gradient allowed the conveying of the material through the barrel, from the hopper section towards the die, and the production of a filament that kept its shape for coiling, with a diameter of about 1.75 mm.

After extrusion, random parts of the printable filaments were used to extract the loaded-pIgG. This step was performed using dichloromethane to solubilize the PLGA matrix (as described in 'Materials and methods' – section II.4.1.4). PBS was then added to solubilize the pIgG [172]. SEC was carried out to generate data about HMWS and LMWS species (Fig. 46). It was demonstrated that HMWS levels were similar for the different filaments produced with 27.5 ± 0.8% (HME_1), 27.8 ± 1.6% (HME_2) and 26.9 ± 2.2% (HME_3) regardless of the PLGA derivative used. The HMWS level of the pIgG model after the SD step (27.3 ± 1.0%) showed that HME did not promote aggregation. However, the LMWS level drastically increased from 4.7 ± 0.6% (pIgG_SD) to 18.8 ± 1.6% (HME_1) when the HME process was performed at 100 °C (Fig. 46). Moreover, no increase in the LMWS level was observed with either HME_2 or HME_3, using slightly lower process temperatures.

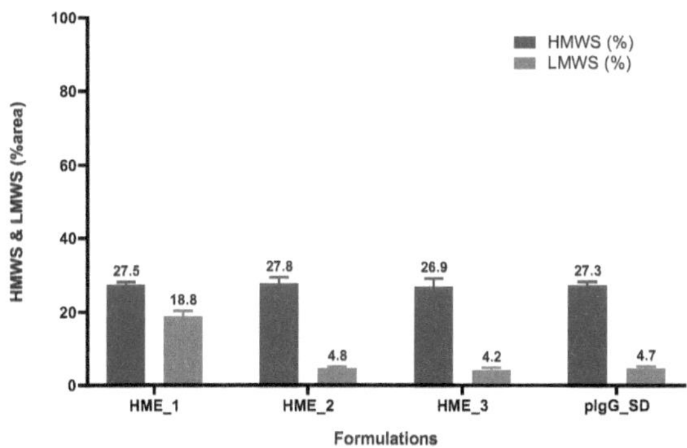

Fig. 46. Comparison of the HMWS and LMWS levels (%) of the pIgG model extracted before SD and after HME for the printable filaments HME_1, HME_2 and HME_3 (n=3, mean ± SD).

All filaments were extruded with a diameter of 1.75 mm, required for the 3D printer. Despite the increase in LMWS levels for HME_1, all the aforementioned filaments (HME_1, HME_2 and HME_3) were used to print 3DP devices to evaluate the stability of the pIgG between the HME and 3DP steps.

II.2 Printing of protein-loaded 3DP devices

HME allowed extruding all the mixtures containing the evaluated PLGA derivatives, plasticizer, stabilizer and pIgG SD powders to produce printable filaments. All the filaments had suitable properties, such as the appropriate diameter of 1.75 mm, resistance and flexibility to be loaded in the 3D printer (MakerBot Replicator 2, NY, USA). DSC evaluations showed that the T_g of the filaments made from HME_1, HME_2 and HME_3 were about 23.5 °C, 24.9 °C and 21.0 °C, respectively (Table 13).

Table 13. Description of the printable filaments characteristics, such as the T_g and pIgG loading percentage, and associated 3DP batch parameters, such as loading and deposition temperatures to print torus devices from HME_1, HME_2 and HME_3, the pIgG loading of a 3DP torus and the weight of devices. All torus devices were printed with dimensions of 5 x 5 x 4 mm (length, width, height) and a layer thickness of 0.1 mm (mean ± SD, n=3).

HME batch number	T_g (°C)	pIgG loading (%)	3DP batch number	Loading temperature (°C)	Deposition temperature (°C)	pIgG loading (%)	Torus weight (mg)
HME_1	23.5	17.3 ± 1.2	3DP_1	130	135	17.8 ± 3.2	41.9 ± 1.3
HME_2	24.9	16.3 ± 2.2	3DP_2	110	113	19.5 ± 4.8	39.7 ± 2.3
HME_3	21.0	16.8 ± 1.6	3DP_3	110	113	15.5 ± 2.5	40.8 ± 2.1

No mass loss at both the loading (i.e. 130 and 110 °C) and deposition temperatures (i.e. 135 °C and 113 °C) was observed on the TGA curves of printable filaments made of the three PLGA (as described in 'Materials and methods' – section II.5.1.2) (Fig. 47). The thermal stability of all PLGA raw material used for this study was demonstrated, and degradation was not expected during the manufacturing of the 3DP devices. However, these results were obtained on filament made of PLGA and not on the filament containing PLGA, plasticizer and pIgG. Further characterization will be required to support the claim that no degradation occurs during both HME and FDM.

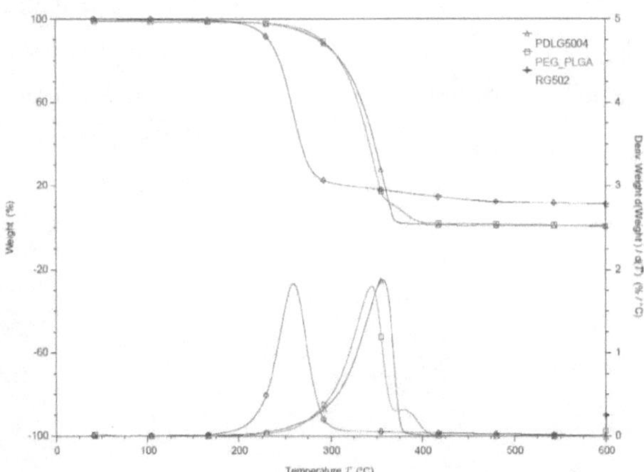

Fig. 47. TGA and DTG curves of the PDLG 5004 (44 kDa), the PEG-PLGA (2 kDa-20 kDa) and the RG502 (7-17 kDa).

A slicing software (ThinkerCAD™, Autodesk® , USA) was used to design a model of a 3DP torus (as described in 'Materials and methods' – section II.3.2) (Fig. 48a). A torus is a donut-shaped circular device which was described in the literature for its zero-order release profile. Indeed, Goyanes et al. reported that surface area to volume ratio was the most important characteristic of a device during the drug release [43].

Investigations on the 3DP torus using printable filaments HME_1, HME_2 and HME_3 were carried out using a MakerBot® Replicator 2 3D printer (MakerBot® Industries, USA). Although this printer has been widely used to produce devices using conventional thermoplastic polymers (e.g. PLA, PVA), some adaptations of standard configurations (e.g. deposition temperature) were performed to print our devices.

The loading temperature was fixed according to the ability of the filaments to be loaded into the 3D printer. Despite the low T_g of printable filaments, the loading temperature was higher than that of the T_{HME} due to the short area/residence time allowed for the melting of the material. Moreover, although the filaments were pushed out by the screws during HME, they had to flow during the printing. It was observed that HME_1 may be loaded at a temperature of 130 °C and both HME_2 and HME_3 at 110 °C.

The difference between the loading temperature and the deposition temperature was that the former reduced the viscosity to promote the flow through the nozzle but was not high enough for the adhesion on the build platform and between successive layers. The latter temperatures were set at 135 °C and 113 °C to print the torus (Fig. 48). Moreover, the fan power was reduced to 10% and first layer was built using a deposition speed of 1 mm/s. Using these parameters, the robustness of the printing was evaluated through the potential variation of the weight of 3DP torus (Table 13). It was observed that the selected deposition temperatures (i.e. 135 °C and 113 °C) allowed the printing of toruses with a similar and reproducible weight of about 40 mg (data not shown). To our knowledge, this is the first time that 3DP devices have been made of PLGA matrix loaded with pIgG.

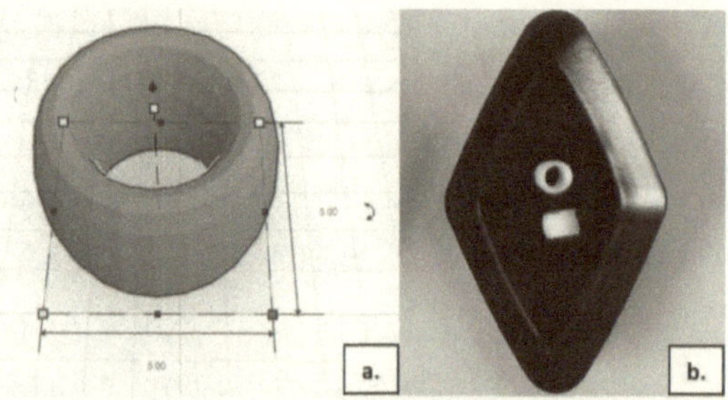

Fig. 48. **a.** Torus device (5 x 5 x 4 mm (length x width x height)) designed with TinkerCad™, **b.** 3DP torus (3DP_3) printed using a MakerBot Replicator 2.

Extraction of the pIgG from the 3DP torus was performed to evaluate the percentage of both HMWS and LMWS (Fig. 49). The HMWS levels of 3DP_1 (8.3 ± 5.9%) were lower than those observed with the 3DP_2 (29.7 ± 5.2%) and 3DP_3 (26.1 ± 1.5%). However, the printable filament HME_1 used to print 3DP_1 was characterized with an HMWS level of 27.5 ± 0.8% (Fig. 46). This unexpected decrease of HMWS could be attributed to the high temperature (i.e. 135 °C) that was used to print 3DP_1 with the HME_1. The denaturation of the pIgG may lead to the formation of insoluble aggregates which were not recovered after the extraction process. However, this was not observed for the other samples, probably due to the use of lower temperatures. The LMWS levels confirmed that 135 °C was clearly deleterious for the pIgG, with a fragmentation percentage that reached 39.1 ± 1.5% (Fig. 49). In contrast, the LMWS levels of 3DP_2 and 3DP_3 were 5.2 ± 0.2% and 5.3 ± 0.6%, respectively. These results were slightly higher than those observed after HME (Fig. 49).

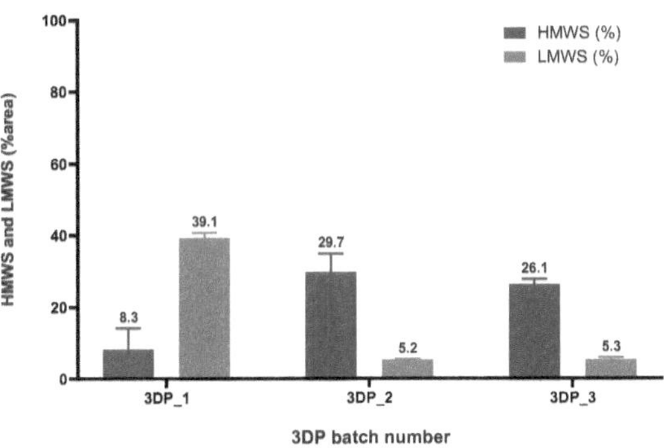

Fig. 49. HMWS and LMWS levels after pIgG extraction from the 3DP torus 3DP_1, 3DP_2 and 3DP_3 (n=3, mean ± SD).

Drug loadings were assessed on the 3DP toruses (as described in 'Materials and methods' – section II.4.1.1b). The BCA results showed loadings lower than the theoretical loading of 20% (w/w) (Table 13). The variability of the loading may be typically due to a lack of homogeneity in the printable filaments. Indeed, it was demonstrated that loadings in printable filaments were lower than those observed after the printing.

The low residence time through the print head led to high degradation levels when high temperatures (i.e. 135 °C) were used. These results showed that PDLG_5004 (HME_1, 3DP_1) was not adapted for this purpose due to the required higher processing temperatures. Overall, PLGA with an inherent viscosity of 0.2 dL/g and an M_w of about 20 kDa were suitable for further investigations (e.g. dissolution testing).

Finally, the release profiles of the melt-encapsulated pIgG model were evaluated on the 3DP toruses (3DP_2 and 3DP_3). It was demonstrated that the burst effect, evaluated after 24h, was higher with 3DP_2 (71.4 ± 3.5%) (Fig. 50) in comparison with that from 3DP_3, which released 21.8 ± 1.7% of the pIgG within 24h. The release after 3 weeks of dissolution reached 84.9 ± 1.5% and 63.3 ± 5.9% with 3DP_2 and 3DP_3, respectively. The 3DP_2 devices tended to reach a plateau after 1 week, with a slow-release phase within 3 weeks (Fig. 50). The higher release that was observed from the 3DP_2 (PEG-PLGA) may be due to the hydrophilic behaviour of the polymeric matrix as PEG was directly linked to PLGA chains. Although the release was influenced by the high surface area of the torus, 3DP_3 sustained the release of the pIgG over 3 weeks. These results demonstrated the potential of RG502 to be used as a bioresorbable polymer to develop 3DP devices containing a biotherapeutic.

131

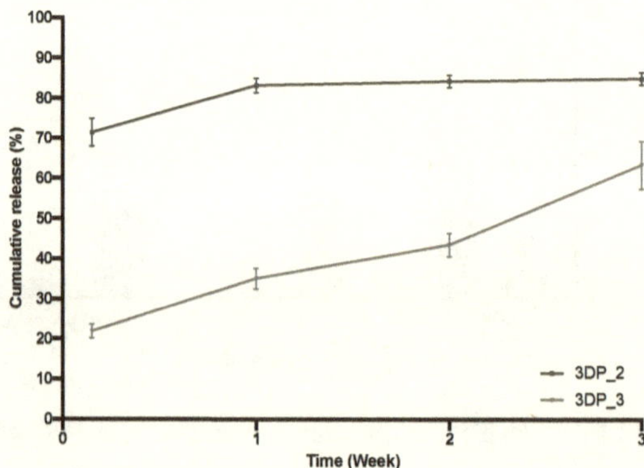

Fig. 50. Dissolution profiles from the 3DP torus 3DP_2 (blue line) and 3DP_3 (red line) containing a pIgG model (n=3, mean ± SD). The release profiles were investigated over 3 weeks and the burst release corresponded to the quantity released within 24h.

II.3 Conclusion

This study was carried out to determine the most suitable PLGA derivatives that may be used to develop 3DP devices containing a pIgG model with a high loading ($\pm$ 20% (w/w)). It represented the first reports of a solid dispersion of an IgG into a biodegradable polymeric matrix using successively HME and FDM. PLGA derivatives characterized by a Mw of about 40 kDa (PDLG_5004) and 20 kDa (RG502) were investigated and 10% (w/w) PEG was added as a plasticizer to decrease the T_g of the polymers. However, a polymeric matrix with a lower Mw (i.e. 20 kDa) allowed the processing temperatures (HME and FDM) to be minimized, which promoted a further thermal stability of the antibody.

Moreover, a PEG-PLGA (2 kDa-20 kDa) was also investigated to evaluate the ability of this diblock copolymer to facilitate both HME and FDM. HMWS and LMWS levels demonstrated the degradation of the pIgG during HME as well as 3DP when PDLG_5004 was used. PLGA, with an inherent viscosity of 0.2 dL/g, seemed to be the most adapted to produce 3DP torus devices, with a slight increase in both HMWS and LMWS levels. Dissolution tests were performed on 3DP toruses to evaluate the release of the pIgG over time. RG502 showed great potential to sustain its release with a limited burst effect and a release over 3 weeks. This preliminary study showed the ability to produce pIgG-loaded 3DP devices with the opportunity to manage several parameters (e.g. the infill percentage). Further investigations are required to improve the HME and to develop uniform printable filaments.

III. Optimization of the printable filaments using HME

III.1 Introduction

The selection of the raw PLGA was performed during the preliminary study. This study was conducted to develop suitable printable filaments for our purpose. The percentage of plasticizer was considered as well as the optimization of the HME to guarantee a homogeneous dispersion of the pIgG model. Then, the stability of the pIgG was evaluated throughout the successive processes, from SD to 3DP (Figure 43). Finally, dissolution tests were carried out on 3DP devices to evaluate the influence of several printing parameters, such as deposition temperature, layer thickness and infill density, on the release profile of the loaded pIgG. The processing steps and the parameters are displayed in Fig. 51.

Briefly, the pIgG was stabilized using Tre and dried to produce a powder (as described in 'Materials and methods' – section II.1.2a). The pIgG powder was blended with PLGA (RG 502) and 10% (w/w) PEG 2kDa before extrusion. The high loading percentage (20% (w/w)) was calculated according to the polymeric matrix (PLGA and PEG 2kDa). Then, the blend was manually fed into the extruder and using a temperature gradient, a filament of 1.75 mm was obtained and manually coiled (as described in 'Materials and methods' – section II.2.2). Finally, the filament was introduced into the print head and devices were printed using the determined parameters (e.g. deposition temperature) (Fig. 51).

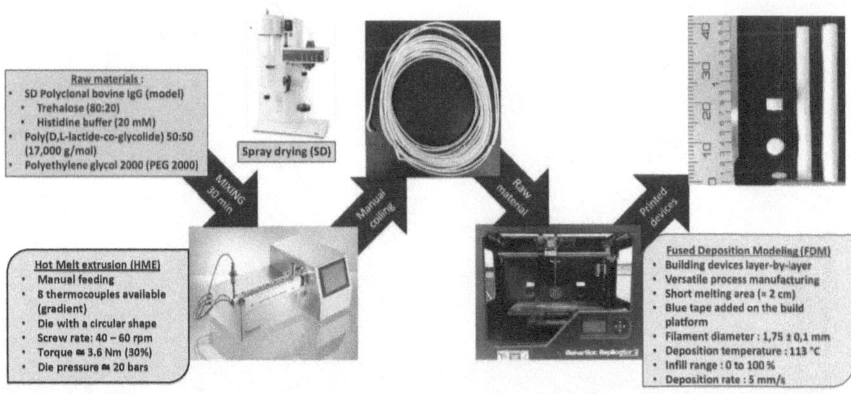

Fig. 51. pIgG-loaded PLGA 3DP devices processing steps overview: spray drying of pIgG in presence of stabilizer, physical mixture of the raw materials, HME processing parameters to produce printable filament, FDM processing parameters to print 3DP devices.

III.2 Results and discussion

III.2.1 Characterizations and optimization of the printable filaments

The thermal properties and thermal stability of all raw materials were assessed using DSC analysis and TGA, respectively (as described in 'Materials and methods' – section II.5.1).

The thermal degradation of the RG502 derivative was conducted using TGA and the associated DTG curves (Fig. 52). The assessment was performed on the extruded filament obtained with the raw polymer and after its blending with all the other components used to improve the processing and enhance the pIgG stability.

The onset degradation temperature of PLGA was higher than those used during HME and 3DP (i.e. 90 and 113-115 °C). The sample containing the pIgG showed a mass loss at temperatures higher than 150 °C (Fig. 52). The plasticization of the RG502 with the PEG 2kDa demonstrated an increase of the thermal stability of the polymer (Fig. 52). The shift of the DTG curve was due to the higher stability of PEG 2kDa through thermal processes. A shift of all DTG curves was observed with PEG 2kDa and pIgG spray-dried powder. Furthermore, the addition of pIgG spray-dried powder seemed to improve the thermal stability but at a lower level than with the use of PEG.

After 3DP, no difference was observed on the curves obtained by TGA. Therefore, it was considered that the printing temperatures that were evaluated did not promote the degradation of the polymer. However, in order to conclude that no degradation occurred at these temperatures, further testing may be required. Indeed, a mass loss was recorded during TGA but no information about the chemical modifications was provided.

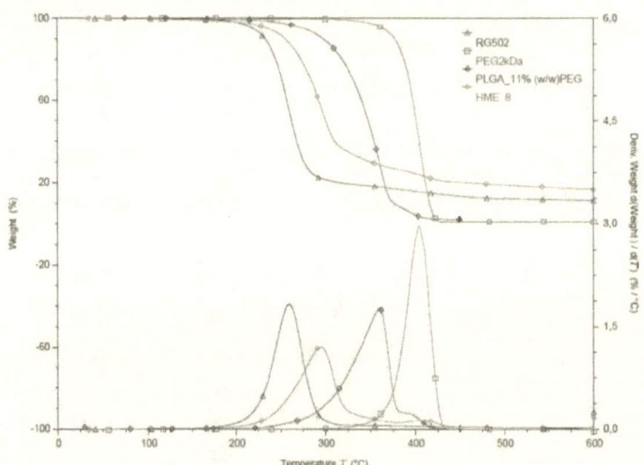

Fig. 52. Comparison of TGA (above) and DTG (below) curves of the RG502, PEG 2kDa, extruded RG502 with 11% (w/w) PEG 2kDa mixture, and printable filament made of RG 502, PEG 2kDa, 20% (w/w) pIgG (the loading percentage of the pIgG was calculated according to the polymeric matrix quantity (i.e. PLGA and PEG 2kDa) (HME_8)).

DSC thermograms of amorphous RG502 showed a T_g of 37.3 ± 0.7 °C (Fig. 53). PEG 2kDa was characterized by a sharp endothermic peak at 52.7 ± 0.2 °C when it was evaluated by DSC (data not shown). The T_g of raw RG 502 shifted to 19.1 ± 0.8 °C using 11% (w/w) of PEG 2kDa (Fig. 53). The T_g of plasticized RG 502 slightly increased up to 21.8 ± 0.5 °C (Fig. 53). No endothermic peak was observed after the HME and 3DP processes, which indicated the homogeneous dispersion of PEG in the PLGA matrix.

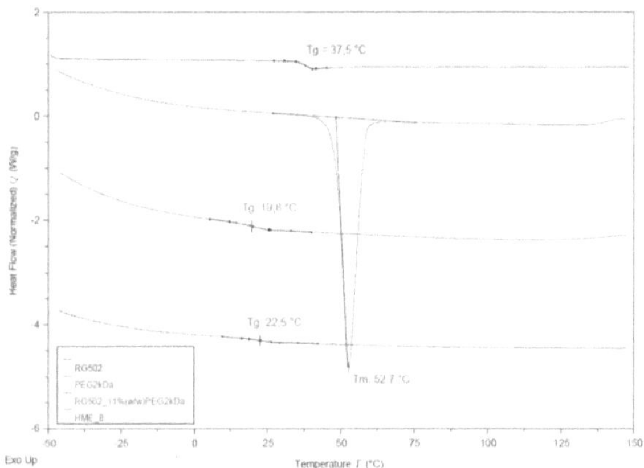

Fig. 53. Comparison of DSC thermograms (first heating cycle) of RG502, PEG 2kDa, RG502 plasticized with 11% (w/w) PEG 2kDa and a printable filament (HME_8) made of RG502, PEG 2kDa and loaded with 20% (w/w) pIgG (the loading percentage of the pIgG was calculated according to the polymeric matrix quantity (i.e. PLGA and PEG 2kDa)).

The influence of the temperature during the storage of the filament was evaluated at -80 °C, 3 °C, 20 °C and 37 °C, with or without the addition of desiccant (Table 14).The addition of desiccant was performed using a hermetically sealed container. Indeed, according to the T_g of our system (i.e. 22 °C), it could be interesting to evaluate its physical stability over time.

No increase in the T_g was observed at -80 °C and 3 °C after 4 weeks of storage. In these conditions, the thermal stability was preserved as these temperatures were lower than the T_g of the filament. In contrast, the T_g increased by up to 32.7 °C after 1 week of storage at 37 °C while an endothermic peak was observed at 48.9 °C on the thermogram (Table 14). This increase was due to the storage temperature, which was higher than the T_g of the filament after HME. Interestingly, at 37 °C, the T_g value decreased over weeks. This may be due to the high mobility of the polymer chains and the presence of moisture, which acted as a plasticizer. However, further evaluations are required to confirm this statement, such as Karl Fisher titration or a TGA. The presence of a desiccant (i.e. silica gel) avoided phase separation between RG502 and PEG 2kDa at 20 °C. Indeed, no endothermic peak was observed after 4 weeks of storage in the presence of a desiccant, while a phase separation occurred after 1 week without desiccant, at 20 °C (Table 14). The miscibility between PEG and polyester was based on physical interaction such as hydrogen bonding or dipole-dipole interactions [209]. Temperatures close to or higher than the T_g of the system led to a separation between PLGA and PEG 2kDa, which was confirmed by the visualization of the T_m of PEG. However, further PEG quantification in the dissolution medium may provide evidence on the phase separation during the dissolution test. In accordance with these results, printable filaments and 3DP devices were stored in a fridge at 3 °C before any further characterizations.

Table 14. Comparison of thermal properties (T_g and T_m) of a filament made of RG502, 11% (w/w) PEG 2kDa and 20% (w/w) pIgG kept at four different storage temperatures (-80 °C, 3 °C, 20 °C and 37 °C), with or without the addition of desiccant (n=1).

Time (week)	- 80 °C				3 °C				20 °C				37 °C			
	No des.		Des.		No des.		Des.		No des.		Des.		No des.		Des.	
	T_g	T_m	T_g	T_m	T_g	T_m	T_g	T_m	T_g	T_m	T_g	T_m	T_g	T_m	T_g	T_m
1	21.9	-	21.7	-	22.3	-	21.9	-	22.4	-	21.3	-	32.7	48.9	35.7	50.0
2	21.3	-	21.6	-	20.8	-	22.5	-	24.6	43.8	22.6	-	31.3	48.7	35.5	50.3
3	21.5	-	21.8	-	21.8	-	22.7	-	25.6	43.2	24.1	-	22.9	48.6	34.3	49.3
4	21.3	-	21.7	-	21.9	-	22.9	-	26.7	43.6	24.2	-	24.4	46.3	35.4	49.1

*(Des.: desiccant (silica gel))

The development of printable filaments based on the use of RG502 was performed at 90 °C (as decribed in 'Materials and methods' – section II.2.2). The temperature was evaluated using the full-barrel length of the Process 11 hot-melt extruder (Thermo Fisher Scientific, USA). However, this temperature needed to be optimized due to the requirement associated with the downstream process (3DP). Indeed, the printable filaments needed to be characterized by a diameter of 1.75 ± 0.05 mm to properly feed the 3D printer [71].

According to the preliminary studies, a plasticizer was required to improve the processability by reducing parameters such torque and die pressure. The addition of PEG 2kDa was previously fixed at 10% w/w compared to the amount of RG502. However, investigations were performed using a percentage of PEG ranged from 10 to 20% (w/w) related to the polymer mass to produce pIgG-loaded printable filaments (Table 15). Indeed, some parts of the previous filaments, which were made with 10% (w/w) of plasticizer, were brittle and a large amount was broken by the gear in the print head of the 3D printer. The increase in the PEG 2kDa content could improve the resistance of the filaments in the printer and minimize the loss of material.

Printable filaments containing a high content of PEG 2kDa (i.e. 20% (w/w) (HME_5) and 15% (w/w) (HME_6)) were investigated (Table 15). Such relatively high amounts of PEG 2kDa led to filaments with high flexibility. However, the viscosity of the melted filaments inside the print head material was too high with 20% (w/w) and 15% (w/w) of PEG 2kDa, with material running out at the die without keeping its rod-shape. It was difficult to guarantee a filament with the appropriate diameter of 1.75 mm. Proportions of 12% (w/w) (HME_7) and 11% (w/w) (HME_8) of 2kDa were also investigated to produce printable filaments (Table 15).

Table 15. Theoretical composition of printable filaments produced using HME batches (% (w/w)) and associated processing parameters such as thermocouple temperature (°C), the yield of the HME and the pIgG loading (%) obtained with BCA assay. (The weight percentage of PEG is related to the polymer mass and the weight percentage of pIgG is related to the polymeric matrix (PLGA and PEG) mass).

HME batch number	Polymer (% w/w)	PEG (% w/w)	Stab. (% w/w)	pIgG (% w/w)	Thermocouple temperature (°C)								Yield (%)	pIgG loading (%)
					#1	#2	#3	#4	#5	#6	#7	Die		
HME_4	66.8	6.7	6.4	20.2	20	40	80	90	90	90	83	73	51.6	17.1 ± 0.4
HME_5	61.0	12.2	6.7	20.1	20	40	80	90	80	90	80	50	63.6	/
HME_6	63.5	9.5	6.7	20.2	20	40	80	90	80	90	80	60	77.1	/
HME_7	65.1	8.1	6.7	20.0	20	40	80	90	90	90	80	75	64.9	/
HME_8	65.8	7.2	6.7	20.2	20	40	80	90	90	90	85	75	68.6	17.2 ± 1.3
HME_9	65.8	7.2	6.7	20.2	20	40	80	90	90	90	85	75	63.1	20.2 ± 0.6
HME_10	65.8	7.2	6.7	20.2	20	40	80	90	90	90	85	75	66.6	19.5 ± 0.3
HME_11	65.8	7.2	6.7	20.2	20	40	80	90	90	90	85	75	66.6	21.4 ± 0.3

*(Stab.: stabilizer (Tre))

The HME was performed on all barrel length using a temperature gradient. Thermocouples 1 and 2 were set at a low temperature (20 °C and 40 °C) to allow convoying the matter towards the subsequent areas and to avoid any overloading of the powder into the hopper. Then, temperatures were increased to reach 90 °C as this is the temperature usually described in literature when RG502 is used [129]. Finally, the last thermocouple and the die were set at 85 °C and 75 °C, respectively (Table 15). Both temperatures were optimized to produce filaments with a diameter of 1.75 mm. The whole process was performed manually, from the feeding to the coiling of the filament (Fig. 51).

A BCA assay was performed to investigate the dispersion of the pIgG inside filaments (as described in 'Materials and methods' – section II.4.1.1b). The theoretical pIgG loading was set at 20% (w/w). The experimental values were lower than the expected loading. Indeed, the loadings were 17.1 ± 0.4% (w/w) and 17.2 ± 1.3% (w/w) with HME_4 and HME_8, respectively (Table 15).

It was demonstrated that pIgG was heterogeneously dispersed into the polymeric matrix when the BCA results of printable filaments and 3DP devices were compared. The HME_8 filament showed a loading of 17.2 ± 1.3%, with a higher variability in comparison with HME_4 (Table 15). However, the 3DP devices using HME_8 as starting material showed an increase in the pIgG loading over the filament length. The first part of the filament was considered as the initial section which emerged from the die. These results demonstrated that pIgG was not homogeneously dispersed in the RG502 matrix. For instance, pIgG loadings evolved from 15.9 ± 0.3% (3DP_6) to 20.2 ± 0.7% (3DP_14) even though the same printable filament (HME_8) was used (Table 16).

Table 16. 3DP batches with the related printable filament and the fixed printing parameters such as deposition temperature (°C), infill percentage (%), layer thickness (mm), the weight of printed cylindrical devices and the pIgG loading (%) determined by BCA assay.

3DP batch number	HME batch number	Deposition temperature (°C)	Infill percentage (%)	Layer thickness (mm)	Weight (mg)	pIgG loading (%)
3DP_4	HME_4	113	50	0.1	43.9 ± 0.7	16.6
3DP_5				0.3	47.7 ± 1.3	16.7
3DP_6	HME_8	113	100	0.1	41.1 ± 5.0	15.9 ± 0.3
3DP_7		114			44.0 ± 0.9	16.2 ± 0.1
3DP_8		115			39.5 ± 3.9	16.1 ± 0.3
3DP_9		113	100	0.3	45.6 ± 0.9	16.0 ± 0.3
3DP_10		114			42.7 ± 3.2	15.7 ± 0.4
3DP_11		115			43.1 ± 3.9	16.0 ± 0.4
3DP_12		113	50	0.1	42.6 ± 0.8	19.3 ± 0.1
3DP_13		114			44.9 ± 1.4	19.7 ± 0.1
3DP_14		115			48.0 ± 1.1	20.2 ± 0.7
3DP_15		113	50	0.3	47.1 ± 3.5	19.7 ± 0.2
3DP_16		114			42.3 ± 3.3	18.5 ± 0.4
3DP_17		115			49.9 ± 1.0	17.6 ± 0.3

These results may be due to the lack of blending before the HME. It was observed that manual blending (RG502, PEG and pIgG powder) with a mortar and a pestle was not effective. The use of a mortar and a pestle led to an increase in the electrostatic charges of the material. The granulometry and the density of RG502, PEG and pIgG powders were also different. The size reduction of the RG502 and PEG using a grinder was carried out after a storage overnight at 37 °C. The roughly ground RG502, PEG and spray-dried pIgG powder were added to a container with stainless steel balls to improve the mixing efficiency. It was determined that a homogeneous physical mixture was reached after 30 minutes in a Turbula® mixer. The handling as well as the powder flow to feed the HME was easier.

This homogeneity was evaluated on two filaments (HME_10 and HME_11) (Table 15). Then, a BCA assay was performed on the entire filament length. The loadings were theoretically set at 20% (w/w) for both HME_10 and HME_11. BCA results confirmed the optimization of the process, with loadings close to the theoretical values with $19.5 \pm 0.3\%$ (HME_10) and $21.4 \pm 0.3\%$ (HME_11) (Table 15). Therefore, the pIgG model was homogeneously dispersed into the RG502 matrix. Overall, the homogeneity of dispersion of the pIgG inside the filaments was maximized by both a well-blended physical mixture and the standard screw configuration.

III.2.2 Development of pIgG-loaded 3DP DDS using FDM technology

The development of pIgG-loaded filaments with a diameter of 1.75 mm was performed. Then, their physicochemical properties were evaluated to ensure their printability.

In accordance with the low T_g of the filaments, the printings were performed in a temperature-controlled room at 20 °C. Indeed, the physical state of the filaments may be quickly modified due to the temperature as their T_g was around 22.5 °C (Fig. 53).

The filaments with a high PEG ratio (HME_5 and HME_6) were unable to be loaded in the printer due to their high flexibility. The filaments were squeezed by the gear during the loading step, then buckling occurred. Hence, the PEG 2kDa content was reduced to 12 and 11% (w/w) (related to the polymer mass). A compromise between brittleness and filament resilience was reached using 11% (w/w) of PEG 2kDa. The presence of 12% (w/w) allowed loading the filaments but all the printing trials done at 113 °C failed. This may be due to thermal conduction and thus the filament was squeezed by the gear during the process. Indeed, the part of the filament above the gear needed to be resilient enough to act as a plunger and push out the material through the nozzle [35]. Further experiments were performed using a quantity of PEG fixed at 11% (w/w) of the RG502.

ThinkerCad™ software (Autodesk®, USA), was used to design the cylindrical shape of the 3DP devices (Fig. 54a). A cylindrical shape was commonly reported in the development of IDDS. Indeed, the development of implantable devices has been mainly performed using HME equipped with circular die geometry, which has led to the production of rod-shaped implants [129,130]. Recently, Steward et al. developed 3DP implantable devices using the Nexplanon® (etonogestrel, contraceptive implant), a rod-shaped implant marketed by Merck as a reference

[55]. At the early stage of the project, torus devices were designed to use a small amount of polymeric material but high burst release was observed. Consequently, after the selection of the raw polymeric material and according to the purpose of the study, the increase of the size and the evaluation of the sustained release of the pIgG will be evaluated on cylindrical devices. These devices allow to modify the infill density of the shapes which may affect the release properties.

Cylindrical devices were successfully produced using three different deposition temperatures (113 °C, 114 °C and 115 °C). The printing was carried out for 2 minutes per device with a diameter of 4 mm and a height of 3 mm (Fig. 54a). The printing was performed at 1 mm/s to promote adhesion of the first layer on the build platform. Then, it was increased to 5 mm/s to print the other layers. These conditions promoted high resolution of the devices and avoided surface defects (Fig. 54b).

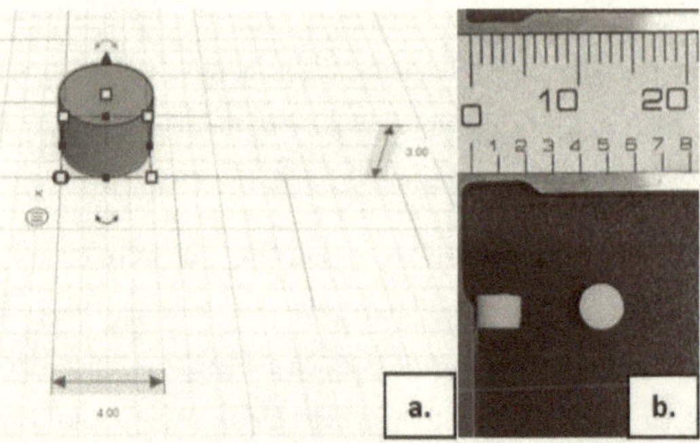

Fig. 54. (a) 3DP cylindrical device (4.0 x 3.0 mm (diameter x length) designed with TinkerCad™, (b) 3DP cylindrical devices (3DP_12) printed using a MakerBot Replicator 2.

III.2.3 Stability of pIgG

The stability of pIgG extracted from both the filament and 3DP devices was assessed and was compared to spray-dried pIgG powder (as described in 'Materials and methods' – section II.4.1.4). The HMWS and LMWS levels were considered to be the critical factor to assess the stability of the pIgG. Indeed, it is commonly accepted that both HMWS and LMWS levels are used to investigate biotherapeutics instabilities [210]. It could be interesting to mention that raw pIgG was already characterized by a high level of both HMWS and LMWS, which were 33.4 ± 2.7% and 5.6 ± 1.2%, respectively.

The printable filament HME_4 was used to produce cylindrical devices printed with two different layer thicknesses (i.e. 0.1 and 0.3 mm) (Table 16). The stability of the pIgG was evaluated and compared after spray-drying, for HME and 3DP. The spray-dried powder was characterized by HMWS and LMWS levels of 27.3 ± 1.0% and 4.7 ± 0.6%, respectively (Fig. 55). These results were lower than those observed with the pIgG raw material. The spray-drying step seemed to increase the stability of the pIgG with the addition of sugar (i.e. Tre). The HMWS level did not increase during the HME and 3DP, with values of 26.7 ± 0.9% (HME_4) and 27.0% (3DP_4) (Fig. 55). However, an increase in LMWS was demonstrated after HME, with a level of 6.8 ± 0.6% (HME_4, Fig. 55).

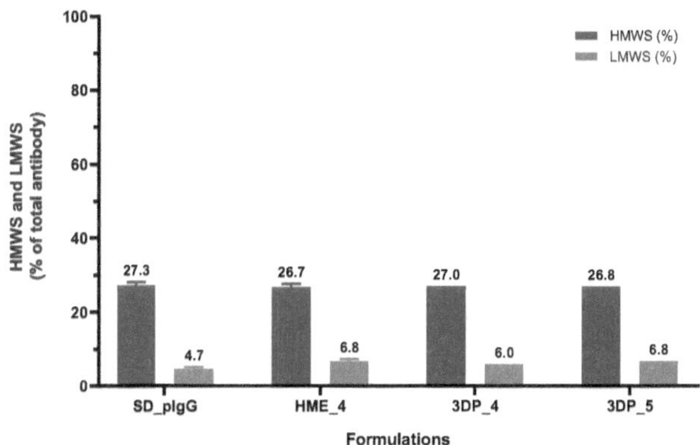

Fig. 55. Comparison of the HMWS and LMWS levels (%) of spray-dried pIgG powder (n=3) and extracted pIgG from both the printable filament produced using HME (HME_4, Table 15) (n=3, mean ± SD) and 3DP devices (3DP_4 (113 °C, 50%, 0.1 mm) and 3DP_5 (113 °C, 50%, 0.3 mm)) (n=1) (Table 16).

A similar evaluation was then performed on printable filament containing 11% (w/w) of PEG (HME_8, Table 12). The HME_8 filament was used to produce 3DP devices at three different deposition temperatures (113 °C, 114 °C, 115 °C). HMWS and LMWS levels were evaluated on printed devices 3DP_6, 3DP_7 and 3DP_9 (Table 16). The HMWS and LMWS levels of spray-dried powders were $28.6 \pm 0.2\%$ and $5.3 \pm 0.4\%$, respectively (Fig. 56). The instability of the pIgG over the manufacturing steps was evaluated in comparison with the spray-dried pIgG levels. The HMWS level was not affected by the HME and the printing at 113 °C (3DP_6) and 114 °C (3DP_7) (p-value > 0.05). However, the HMWS level showed a significant increase to $30.6 \pm 1.9\%$ (p-value < 0.05) at 115 °C. In contrast, no significant difference in LMWS levels was observed over the successive processing steps (HME and FDM) in comparison with the spray-dried pIgG powder level. According to these results, the integrity of the pIgG may be preserved over successive steps, except when devices were printed at 115 °C. Increasing the temperatures led to temperatures close to the T_g of Tre (~ 120 °C). Therefore, the stabilization effect of the glassy matrix of Tre may be less effective at 115 °C in comparison with the lower printing temperatures (113 and 114 °C).

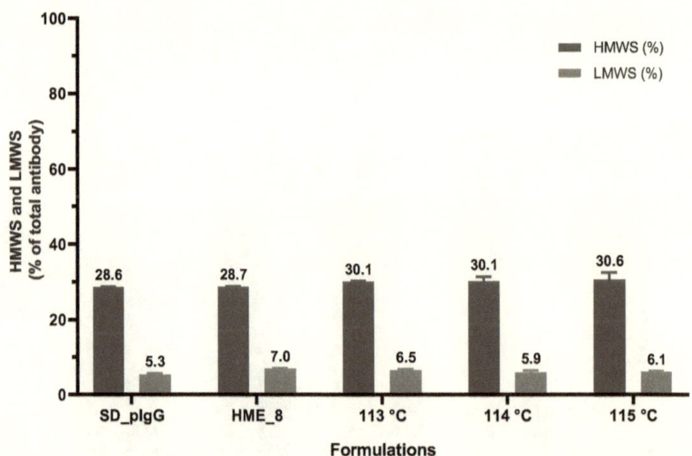

Fig. 56. Comparison of the HMWS and LMWS levels (%) of the spray-dried pIgG powder, the extracted pIgG model from printable filament produced using HME (HME_8, Table 15) and the pIgG model extracted from 3DP devices printed at 113 °C (3DP_6), 114 °C (3DP_8) and 115 °C (3DP_9) (Table 16).

III.2.4 Dissolution study

The 3DP was able to produce devices using a plethora of parameters. It was reported that the release profile of the drug compounds can be modulated with the variation of the infill density [83]. In this study, the influence of the deposition temperature and the layer thickness on the dissolution profile of the loaded pIgG were investigated.

III.2.4.1 Effect of the deposition temperature

It was previously demonstrated that a minimal deposition temperature of 113 °C was required to print the devices. However, it seemed interesting to test other temperatures to investigate their influence on the release profiles. The printable filament HME_8 was used to print devices at 113 °C (3DP_6), 114 °C (3DP_7) and 115 °C (3DP_8) (Table 16).

The release of the pIgG was sustained over 12 weeks (Fig. 57). The preliminary study showed a release over 3 weeks with torus devices (Fig. 50). These results demonstrated that the shape of the devices influenced the release duration and profile. Differences in the release patterns were observed when comparing all 3DP devices. It was demonstrated that the burst effect of the pIgG from 3DP_6 reached 24.2 ± 3.7% after 24h of release, while its release from 3DP_7 and 3DP_8 was 9.2 ± 1.8% and 19.1 ± 2.4%, respectively. A temperature of 113 °C (3DP_6) allowed printing of devices but the viscosity of the melted polymer was potentially too low to guarantee cohesion between the layers. Therefore, the porosity at the surface of 3DP_6 would be higher than that of 3DP_7 and 3DP_8. In general, there was a faster release within 1 week observed with all profiles. For instance, the cumulated release of 3DP_7 increased from 9.1 ± 1.8% (burst effect) to 29.1 ± 7.8 % (Fig. 57). This increase may be due to the presence of pore formers such as PEG 2kDa and Tre, which may increase the release of the pIgG [102]. After 1 week, the release was slowed down on all dissolution profiles. This slowdown may be due to the swelling of the PLGA matrix, which decreased the porosity of the systems.

It was previously reported that the erosion of rod-shaped HME implants made of PLGA started after 4 weeks and an increase in the release of a loaded protein model (i.e. BSA) was observed [129]. However, a low release phase was observed over 8 weeks with the BSA.

From week 1 to week 8, it was shown that the cumulative release of pIgG reached only 69.0 ± 0.2% (3DP_6), 46.5 ± 6.3% (3DP_7) and 53.9 ± 5.8% (3DP_8). After 8 weeks, a maximum release of 99.5 ± 0.6%, 76.8 ± 3.5% and 71.1 ± 6.5% was reached with 3DP_6, 3DP_7 and 3DP_8, respectively. Overall, the release profiles of 3DP devices were compared using the similarity factor (f2). It was observed that 3DP_6 had a different release profile from 3DP_7 and 3DP_8 as the f2 values were lower than 50 with 42.6 and 48.1, respectively. The f2 value of devices 3DP_7 and 3DP_8 was 64.9 and demonstrated similarity between the curves.

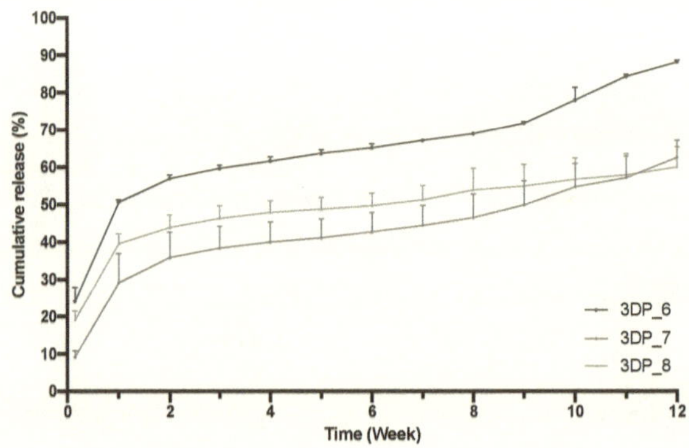

Fig. 57. Influence of the deposition temperature (from 113 °C to 115 °C) on the release profiles of pIgG-loaded 3DP cylindrical devices printed with an infill density of 100% and a layer thickness of 0.1 mm: 3DP_6 (113 °C), 3DP_7 (114 °C) and 3DP_8 (115 °C) (n=3, mean ± SD).

The HMWS levels were evaluated during the dissolution test of 3DP_6, 3DP_7 and 3DP_8 (Fig. 58). The levels observed after the burst effect were the highest after 10 weeks, with 23.9 ± 5.8% (3DP_6), 24.0 ± 0.5% (3DP_7) and 21.4 ± 8.5% (3DP_8). Surprisingly, these values were lower than expected according to the values previously shown after extraction of the pIgG from the 3DP devices. For instance, 3DP_7 was characterized by an HMWS level of 32.1 ± 0.8% (Fig. 58). The difference between these values may be due to the degradation of the pIgG during the HME and 3DP. Indeed, it has been reported that noncovalent aggregation of BSA occurred during HME at 90 °C [129]. Therefore, adding an additional process using heat such as with 3DP may have led to an increase in the instabilities and thermally driven chemical reactions such as acylation [102]. It was estimated that only noncovalent aggregates were characterized by SEC, which could explain these results. In contrast, the increase in the HMWS levels from week 6 to week 10 was due to the erosion of the matrix and the acidic microenvironment created by the progressive hydrolysis of PLGA.

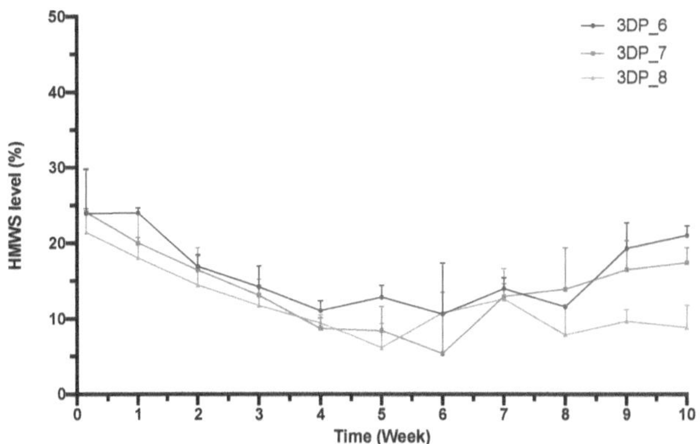

Fig. 58. Comparison of HMWS levels (%) over the dissolution test (pIgG released from polymeric matrix) for 3DP cylindrical devices printed using three different temperatures: 3DP_6 (113 °C), 3DP_7 (114 °C) and 3DP_8 (115 °C) (n=3, mean ± SD).

The evaluation of LMWS levels was also performed during the dissolution test of 3DP_6, 3DP_7 and 3DP_8. As previously mentioned, the pIgG was thermally degraded during the 3DP. The LMWS levels confirmed the degradation, with an increase in the value over weeks (Fig. 59). It was reported that fragmentation mainly occurs with the acidification of the dissolution medium or high temperatures [153]. In this case, the main degradation pathway was due to the high temperatures (i.e. 113 to 115 °C) during the 3DP.

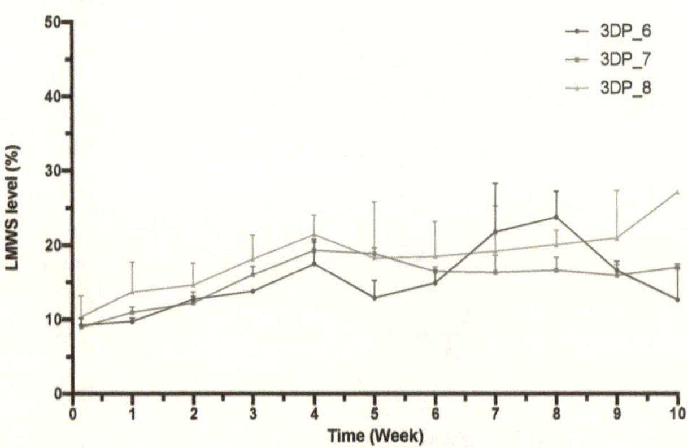

Fig. 59. Comparison of LMWS levels (%) over the dissolution test (pIgG released from polymeric matrix) for 3DP devices printed using three different temperatures: 3DP_6 (113 °C), 3DP_7 (114 °C) and 3DP_8 (115 °C) (n=3, mean ± SD).

III.2.4.2 Influence of the layer thickness

The layer thickness was described to be a printing parameter which modifies the resolution of the printed devices. A decrease in the layer thickness (i.e. 0.1 mm) was reported to improve the resolution [30]. FDM is recognised as a 3DP technique with a low resolution which is unable to produce fine structures [48]. However, it could be interesting to investigate this parameter to modify or customize the release of the dispersed pIgG. In the literature, the use of standard resolution (i.e. 0.2 mm) is usually described. When other thicknesses were used (i.e. 0.1 mm and 0.3 mm), no evaluation was done on their influence on the drug release [54,88,211]. The use of layer thicknesses of 0.1 and 0.3 mm allowed the influence of this parameter on the release profile to be evaluated properly.

In our case, devices were printed with two different layer thicknesses of 0.1 mm and 0.3 mm using a deposition temperature set at 114 °C and an infill density of 100% (Table 16). The dissolution profile of both printed devices was evaluated (Fig. 60). The burst effect was increased up to 21.2 ± 8.1% (3DP_10) when the layer thickness was set at 0.3 mm. The release from 3DP_10 was faster than that observed with 3DP_7, with a cumulative release of 91.0 ± 3.5% and 62.6 ± 4.6%, respectively. However, both profiles were statistically similar with an f2 value of 52.5.

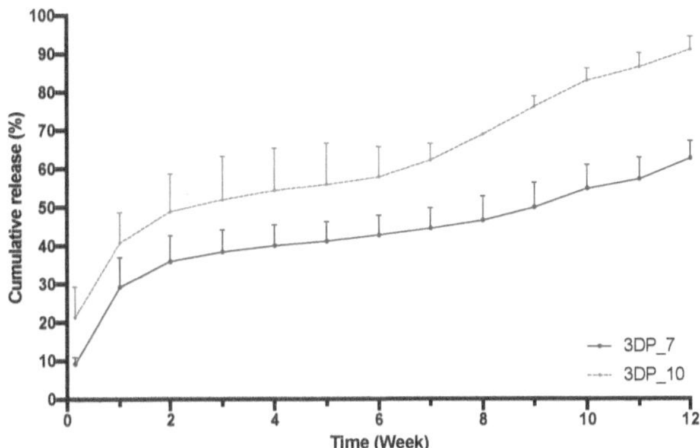

Fig. 60. Influence of the layer thickness (0.1 mm and 0.3 mm) on the release profiles of pIgG-loaded 3DP devices printed with an infill density of 100% and a deposition temperature set at 114 °C: 3DP_7 (0.1 mm) and 3DP_10 (0.3 mm) (n=3, mean ± SD).

Interestingly, the comparison between both layer thicknesses at 115 °C showed closer dissolution profiles and led to an increase in the f2 value up to 67.1. The burst effects of 3DP_8 (19.1 ± 2.4%) and 3DP_11 (12.3 ± 6.2%) were not different (Fig. 61). The release profile of 3DP_11 was slightly faster than that observed from 3DP_8.

These results may confirm that the deposition temperature may be too low to promote a well-defined structure without defect. The release of the pIgG from the devices was mainly driven by the surface area to volume ratio as described in literature [43]. Therefore, 3DP devices with similar dimensions (4 x 3 mm) and infill densities (100%) were expected to be similar in terms of release profiles, irrespective of the layer thickness.

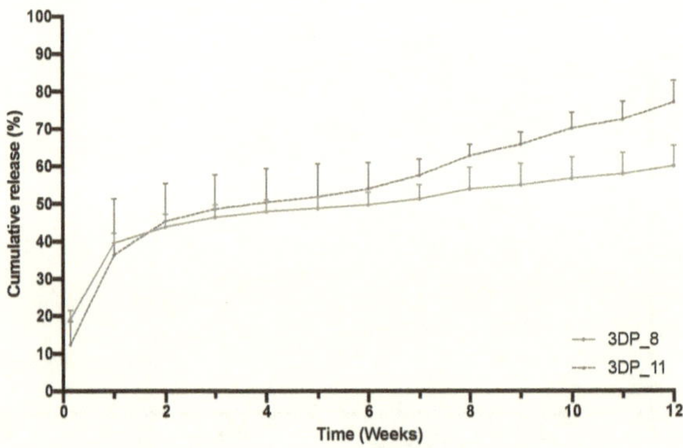

Fig. 61. Influence of the layer thickness (0.1 mm and 0.3 mm) on the release profiles of pIgG-loaded 3DP devices printed with an infill density of 100% and with a deposition temperature set at 115 °C: 3DP_8 (0.1 mm) and 3DP_11 (0.3 mm) (n=3, mean ± SD).

III.2.4.3 Influence of the infill density

Numerous authors have reported the influence of the infill density of the printed devices on the release patterns [37,62]. The flexibility of the devices and the ability to modulate the dose could be achieved by adjusting the infill density. The infill can be changed from 0% to 100%, which correspond to a hollow device or a fully solid device, respectively [212]. Here, devices were printed with two different infill densities (50% (3DP_13) and 100% (3DP_7)) (Table 16).

The release profiles of the pIgG showed a higher burst effect when a greater infill percentage was fixed. Indeed, the percentage of release reached $5.6 \pm 0.6\%$ and $9.2 \pm 1.8\%$ from 3DP_13 and 3DP_7, respectively (Fig. 62). This may be due to the degradation of the surface of the devices, which was similar for all. Indeed, the infill percentage was modulated but the external surface was fixed at two shell layers as a default setting. The slight difference could be explained by the similarity between both devices. However, no difference was observed after 12 weeks of dissolution. The release of pIgG from 3DP_7 was slower than observed with 3DP_13 in terms of cumulative release over weeks. This may be due to the water uptake in 3DP_13, which was facilitated due to its low density. Indeed, no lag phase was observed with 3DP_13, which was characterized by the continuous dissolution and diffusion of the pIgG from the polymeric matrix over time.

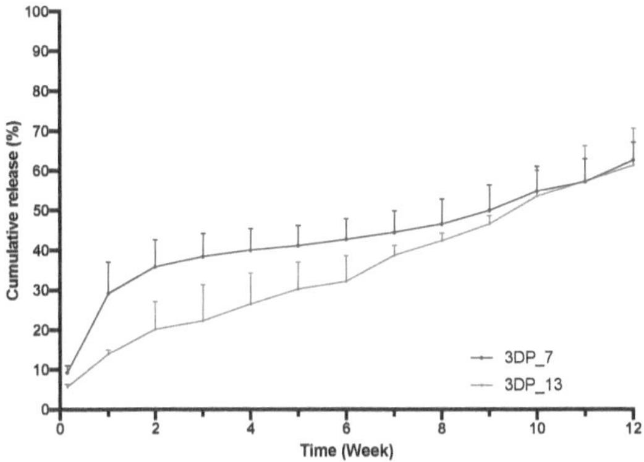

Fig. 62. Influence of the infill density (50% and 100%) on the release profiles of pIgG-loaded 3DP devices printed with a layer thickness of 0.1 mm and a deposition temperature set at 114 °C: 3DP_7 (100%) and 3DP_13 (50%) (n=3, mean ± SD).

The release of the drug from the PLGA-based system is mainly carried out by erosion and diffusion of the drug through the porous network. However, the swelling and the degradation of the PLGA led to hydrodynamic modification of the system overtime. Both mechanisms influence the formation of a porous network, leading to potential modification of the dissolution profile of a loaded drug.

III.2.4.4 Thermal properties of the devices during the dissolution test

DSC thermograms of 3DP devices in dissolution medium showed the evolution of the T_g after 8 consecutive weeks (Fig. 63). Devices were removed from the dissolution medium and dried under vacuum before analysis by DSC. It was showed that the T_g increased from 20.6 °C to 38.8 °C within 3 weeks. This may be due to the release of PEG in the dissolution medium. The T_g of the system was lower than temperature of the dissolution medium, which was set at 37 °C. The mobility of polymeric chains rapidly increased at 37 °C, increasing potential phase separation issues. In accordance with the low amount of PEG into the PLGA matrix, the phase separation occurred within 3 weeks. After this, the T_g slowly decreased to 28.8 °C after 8 weeks of dissolution. The hydrolysis of the RG502 derivatives may lead to a decrease in the T_g after 4 weeks.

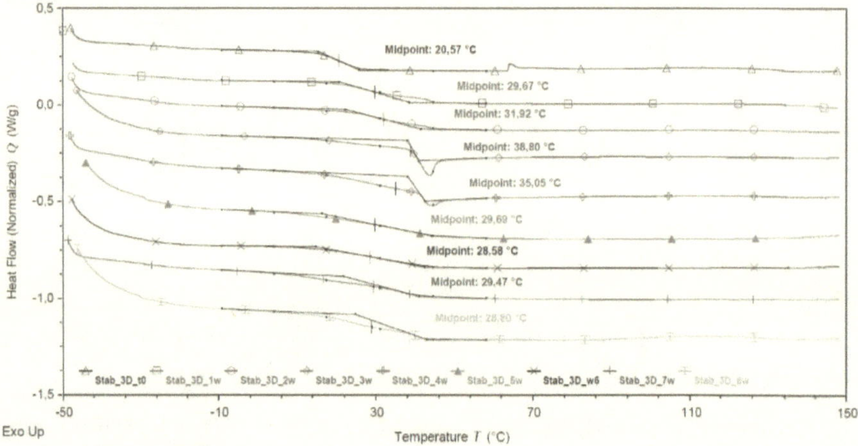

Fig. 63. DSC thermograms (first heating cycle) shown the variation of Tg of pIgG-loaded 3DP devices during a dissolution test over 8 weeks.

III.2.4.5 Scanning electron microscopy

SEM pictures were taken of 3DP cylindrical devices after 8 weeks of dissolution (as described in 'Materials and methods' – section II.6) (Fig. 64). As previously mentioned, the 3DP devices were removed from the dissolution medium and dried under vacuum before analysis by DSC. The reference 3DP device showed a nearly poreless surface and well-defined layers at the start of the dissolution test in accordance with fixed parameters (113 °C and 0.1 mm of layer thickness). It was observed that degradation of the surface occurred after 1 week of dissolution. Indeed, some defects were observed on the surface of the devices (i.e. pores and cracks) (Fig. 64b). These cracks could be correlated with the diffusion of the medium into the system. The degradation continued to occur, and larger cracks were identified after 3 weeks (Fig. 64c). Deformation and swelling of the device should occur after 4 weeks. At this stage, the layers of the devices were no longer distinguishable (Fig. 64d). After 8 weeks of dissolution, the lateral surface of the cylinder appeared uniformly porous (Fig. 64e). Nevertheless, the drying step, which was performed under vacuum, could be involved in the appearance of surface defects. The release of hydrophilic compounds such as PEG 2kDa over time tended to increase the brittleness of the PLGA matrix.

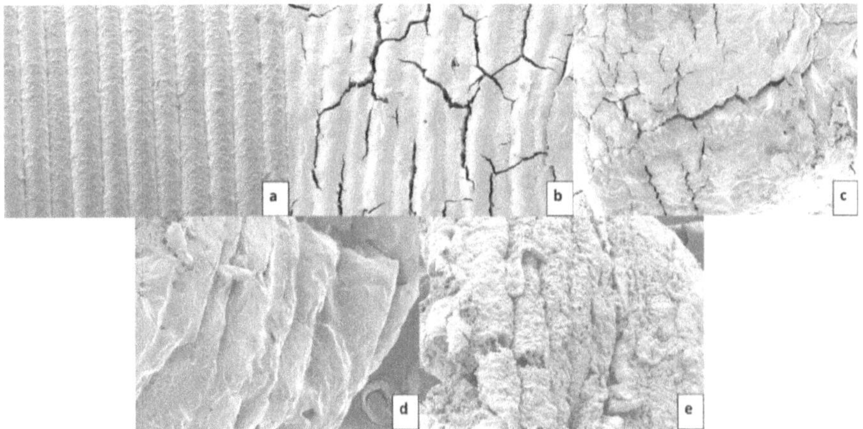

Fig. 64. SEM micrographs of 3DP cylindrical devices (4 mm x 3 mm (diameter x height), 50% infill, layer thickness of 0.1 mm, 113 °C) over time during dissolution study with: (**a**) the reference device after 3DP, (**b**) the sample after 1 week, (**c**) after 3 weeks, (**d**) after 4 weeks and (**e**) after 8 weeks in dissolution medium (100x magnification).

These observations demonstrated that the diffusion of the medium and the subsequent degradation of the cylindrical surface occurred rapidly. The diffusion of the medium was promoted by the formation of pores, which influenced the release of the pIgG. It could be interesting to enhance our knowledge on the degradation of RG502 matrix over time using GPC measurements.

III.3 Conclusion

The formulation and the development of 3DP cylindrical devices containing a model of pIgG with a high loading of 20% (w/w) was achieved via FDM technology. Printable filaments were optimized to reach the physical behaviour required to be printed with a PEG content set at 11% (w/w) of RG502. The HME process was improved to guarantee a reproducible homogenous dispersion of pIgG at 20% (w/w) into the filaments.

The influence of different parameters (i.e. pIgG loading, HME and FDM temperatures, infill density) on the release of the pIgG were investigated during this study. A polymeric matrix made of RG502 allowed producing filaments at 90 °C. Despite the low viscosity of the polymer, 3DP was performed at a minimum temperature of 113 °C. It was shown that the deposition temperature influenced the release profile of the pIgG and that 113 °C led to a high burst effect and a fast release of the pIgG over time. Devices printed at 114 and 115 °C demonstrated slower release of the pIgG over 12 weeks. However, the release of pIgG was characterized by a high level of LMWS even after 24h of release. This was mainly related to the high printing temperature.

This study demonstrated the ability to produce pIgG-loaded filaments to be printed using FDM technology. Based on these results, the feasibility of printing mAb-loaded 3DP devices will be assessed in the next chapter. Further characterizations in terms of stability during the process and binding capacities will be also investigated.

Part III – Development of PLGA mAb-loaded 3D-printed implantable devices using fused-deposition modelling technology

I.   Introduction

In the previous section, the feasibility of using HME and FDM to produce pIgG-loaded 3DP devices was demonstrated. The formulation of the printable filaments was optimized and the influence of different printing parameters (i.e. temperature, layer thickness and infill density) on the release profile of the loaded pIgG was evaluated.

The novelty of this work was to investigate the ability of FDM to print sustained-release mAb-loaded DDS. Indeed, to our knowledge, there is no published paper describing biotherapeutic-loaded DDS made by FDM. This is probably because HME and FDM are both based on the use of relatively high temperatures, which may be deleterious for the mAb. Therefore, it was necessary to select judiciously the type of thermoplastic polymer (i.e. PLGA RG502) to be used and to optimize the manufacturing parameters of both techniques. The formulation of the mAb was optimized by testing several stabilizers (i.e. Suc, Tre, HP-β-CD, Sor, Inu, Leu) at three different mAb:stabilizer ratios, such as 1.5:1, 2.0:1 and 2.5:1. This was done to obtain a DDS that could allow maintaining the stability and the affinity of the loaded mAb after the process.

Moreover, after the 3DP of the mAb-loaded DDS, it was interesting to evaluate the stability of the mAb in terms of physical state, quantification, dissolution profile and binding capacity over 6 months.

II.   Results and discussion

Initially, the mAb solution was formulated with different stabilizers. These solutions were spray dried to produce mAb-loaded powders (as described in 'Materials and methods' – section II.1.2 b). Indeed, it was necessary to stabilize mAb in solid state to increase its stability and to facilitate handling during further processing. Then, a physical mixture of mAb-loaded spray-dried powder, RG502 and PEG was extruded using HME to produce printable filaments (as described in 'Materials and methods' – section II.2.2). These printable filaments were used to feed the 3DP printer and to print our devices (as described in 'Materials and methods' – section II.3.3). The selection of the optimal formulation was carried out by evaluating mAb integrity after each processing step (SD, HME, 3DP). The *in vitro* evaluations (dissolution test and binding capacity) were performed on the selected mAb formulation and a stability study was performed over 6 months.

II.1 Preliminary study on raw materials and printable filaments

The thermal properties, including degradation temperature, of all raw materials were assessed using TGA and DSC analysis, respectively.

The TGA thermograms of the spray-dried mAb powder (SD_19, mAb:Tre-Leu ratio 2.0:1 (Table 17)) showed a slight weight loss at 100 °C (Fig. 65). Such decrease could be attributed to the residual moisture content in the spray-dried mAb powder. Indeed, the mean residual moisture in the spray-dried powders was found to be $3.4 \pm 0.8\%$. No further drying was performed to reduce the residual moisture, but the storage of the mAb-loaded spray-dried powders was carried out in a desiccator under vacuum. It may be interesting to compare these results using Karl Fisher titration in further investigations. A second weight loss was observed above 150 °C on all the spray-dried mAb-loaded powders, which led to the degradation of the compound (Fig. 65). Therefore, it seemed that the mAb-loaded powders could ensure the physical stability of the mAb during both HME and 3DP, which were performed at maximal temperatures of 90 °C and 105 °C, respectively. The investigation of the secondary and the tertiary structure of mAb should also be done but was out of the scope of this study. In comparison with the TGA thermograms, evaluation of the mAb structure may demonstrate chemical degradation.

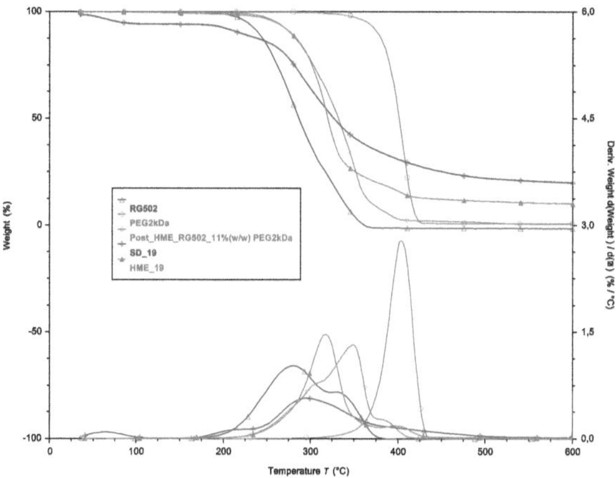

Fig. 65. TGA and associated DTG curves of RG502, PEG 2kDa, extruded RG502 and PEG mixture, spray-dried mAb powder (SD_19), and extruded printable filament (HME_19), which were selected to illustrate the thermal degradation.

Table 17. Theoretical composition of evaluated mAb formulations for spray-dried batches (% w/V), solid composition of spray-dried powders (% w/w) and the yield of the SD process (%), printable filaments produced using HME batches (% w/w) with the yield of the process (%) (Process-11, ThermoFisher Scientific, USA) and associated 3DP batches with layer thickness of 0.1 mm and 0.3 mm and differing infill percentages (% (v/v)) (Hyrel 30M sytem, Hyrel, USA). Histidine buffer was used in the mAb solution before SD. The excipient 'Leu' will be described later in the text.

SD batch number	Stab.	mAb:stab. ratio	His	Stab.	Leu	mAb	His	Stab.	Leu	mAb	SD yield (%)	HME batch number	RG502 (% w/w)	PEG (% w/w)	Excipient (% w/w)	mAb (% w/w)	HME yield (%)	3DP layer thickness 0.1 mm infill % (v/v) 10	50	100	3DP layer thickness 0.3 mm infill % (v/v) 10	50	100
			Liquid composition (% w/V) - after BE				Solid composition (% w/w) - after spray drying																
SD_1		1.5:1	0.2	5.1	-	8.0	1.7	38.3	-	60.0	80.6	HME_1	60.1	6.6	13.3	20.0	44,6	3DP_1	-	-	3DP_2	-	-
SD_2	Suc	2.0:1	0.2	3.8	-	8.0	1.9	31.4	-	66.7	82.7	HME_2	62.9	6.9	10.1	20.1	39,5	3DP_3	-	-	3DP_4	-	-
SD_3		2.5:1	0.2	3.2	-	8.0	2.1	26.5	-	71.4	88.2	HME_3	64.1	7.1	8.7	20.2	39,8	3DP_5	-	-	3DP_6	-	-
SD_4		1.5:1	0.2	5.1	-	8.0	1.7	38.3	-	60.0	78.4	HME_4	60.1	6.6	13.3	20.0	48,4	3DP_7	-	-	3DP_8	-	-
SD_5	Tre	2.0:1	0.2	3.8	-	8.0	1.9	31.4	-	66.7	84.1	HME_5	62.9	6.9	10.1	20.1	41,5	3DP_9	-	-	3DP_10	-	-
SD_6		2.5:1	0.2	3.2	-	8.0	2.1	26.5	-	71.4	89.7	HME_6	64.1	7.1	8.7	20.2	41,5	3DP_11	-	-	3DP_12	-	-
SD_7		1.5:1	0.2	5.1	-	8.0	1.7	38.3	-	60.0	79.9	HME_7	60.1	6.6	13.3	20.0	44,3	3DP_13	-	-	3DP_14	-	-
SD_8	Sor	2.0:1	0.2	3.8	-	8.0	1.9	31.4	-	66.7	81.6	HME_8	62.9	6.9	10.1	20.1	44,4	3DP_15	-	-	3DP_16	-	-
SD_9		2.5:1	0.2	3.2	-	8.0	2.1	26.5	-	71.4	87.4	HME_9	64.1	7.1	8.7	20.2	42,9	3DP_17	-	-	3DP_18	-	-
SD_10		1.5:1	0.2	5.1	-	8.0	1.7	38.3	-	60.0	99.1	HME_10	60.1	6.6	13.3	20.0	43,6	3DP_19	-	-	3DP_20	-	-
SD_11	Inu	2.0:1	0.2	3.8	-	8.0	1.9	31.4	-	66.7	102.8	HME_11	62.9	6.9	10.1	20.1	42,1	3DP_21	-	-	3DP_22	-	-
SD_12		2.5:1	0.2	3.2	-	8.0	2.1	26.5	-	71.4	93.1	HME_12	64.1	7.1	8.7	20.2	40,9	3DP_23	-	-	3DP_24	-	-
SD_13		1.5:1	0.2	5.1	-	8.0	1.7	38.3	-	60.0	103.5	HME_13	60.1	6.6	13.3	20.0	62,2	3DP_25	-	-	3DP_26	-	-
SD_14	HP-β-CD	2.0:1	0.2	3.8	-	8.0	1.9	31.4	-	66.7	100.8	HME_14	62.9	6.9	10.1	20.1	45,1	3DP_27	-	-	3DP_28	-	-
SD_15		2.5:1	0.2	3.2	-	8.0	2.1	26.5	-	71.4	106.1	HME_15	64.1	7.1	8.7	20.2	39,7	3DP_29	-	-	3DP_30	-	-
SD_16	Suc	2.0:1	0.2	3.8	-	8.0	1.9	31.4	-	66.7	80.3	HME_16	69.4	7.6	7.6	15.3	67,6	3DP_31	-	-	3DP_32	3DP_33	3DP_34
SD_17	Suc-Leu	2.0:1	0.2	3.2	0.6	8.0	1.9	26.4	5	66.7	84.1	HME_17	69.4	7.6	7.6	15.3	65,5	-	-	-	3DP_35	3DP_36	3DP_37
SD_18	Tre	2.0:1	0.2	3.8	-	8.0	1.9	31.4	-	66.7	80.8	HME_18	69.4	7.6	7.6	15.3	65,9	3DP_38	-	-	3DP_39	3DP_40	3DP_41
SD_19	Tre-Leu	2.0:1	0.2	3.2	0.6	8.0	1.9	26.4	5	66.7	83.8	HME_19	69.4	7.6	7.6	15.3	68,9	-	-	-	3DP_42	3DP_43	3DP_44
SD_20	Tre-Leu	2.0:1	0.2	3.2	0.6	8.0	1.9	26.4	5	66.7	85.1	HME_20	69.4	7.6	7.6	15.3	65,8	-	-	-	-	-	3DP_45
SD_21	Tre-Leu	2.0:1	0.2	3.2	0.6	8.0	1.9	26.4	5	66.7	85.3	HME_21	69.4	7.6	7.6	15.3	59,0	-	-	-	-	-	3DP_46

*(Stab.: stabilizer, His.: histidine buffer, Leu.: further excipient)

In addition, the physical degradation temperature of raw RG502 was around 175 °C (Fig. 65). Moreover, it was observed that no apparent weight loss appeared under 200 °C for raw PEG and for the extruded filaments loaded with mAb. No residual moisture was observed in RG502 and PEG raw materials. These results confirmed that all raw materials seemed stable and may be processed according to the temperatures in both HME and FDM (90 °C and 105 °C, respectively). However, only the mass loss was characterized using TGA. Other methods were required to state the mAb stability, such as SEC and binding capacity.

DSC analyses were carried out to evaluate the influence of the addition of PEG and mAb-loaded spray-dried powder on the T_g of the thermoplastic polymer RG502 (Fig. 66). Indeed, as the aim of this work was to develop mAb-loaded 3DP DDS, the T_g should be as low as possible to decrease the temperature of the different processes (HME, 3DP), and avoid the potential degradation of the biotherapeutic as a consequence.

The T_g of RG502 was found to be 38.0 ± 0.7 °C, which was consistent with data already described in the literature [213] (Fig. 66). PEG was characterized by a sharp endothermic peak at 52 °C. The T_g of RG502 decreased to 21.8 ± 0.4 °C when 11% (w/w) PEG and spray-dried powder were added during HME (Fig. 66). Such decrease in the T_g, in addition to the loss of the sharp melting peak of PEG, demonstrated that mAb-loaded spray-dried powder and PEG were properly dispersed in the molten polymer matrix [60]. This step was mandatory to ensure the further physical stability of the system before any other investigations. It is widely accepted that miscibility between polymer-polymer, polymer-API or amorphous mixtures of APIs is related to a unique T_g value [214,215].

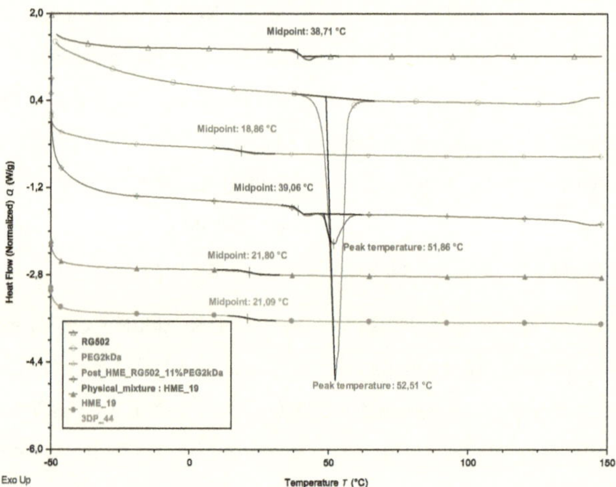

Fig. 66. DSC thermograms (first heating cycle) of RG502, PEG 2kDa, extruded RG502-11% (w/w) PEG mixture, physical mixture of HME_19, extruded printable filament (HME_19) and associated 3DP devices (3DP_44).

II.2 Formulation screening and mAb stability after spray-drying

Stabilizers were selected to maintain mAb integrity during all the manufacturing steps. The main deleterious factor was the relatively high temperatures that were used during both HME and FDM. It is widely accepted that sugars are effective excipients for stabilizing mAb during SD [155]. The solid state improves thermal stress resistance, shear-induced denaturation and surface adsorption instabilities [216]. Unfortunately, there is no universal stabilizer and the choice needs to be adapted to each biotherapeutic according to the stress factors associated with the process [132,140]. The following discussion will focus on the HMWS and LMWS levels which must remain as low as possible. There is no establish criteria on HMWS and LMWS levels but an aggregate level limited to less than 5% in commercial intravenous immunoglobulin product is acceptable according to the World Health Organisation standards [132]. However, this value may be modulated depending on the molecule and the administration route. According to this work and the high process temperatures used, the formulations with the lowest HMWS and LMWS levels were selected for futher experiments.

Suc, Tre, HP-β-CD, Sor and Inu are commonly used in mAb formulations [217–221]. It was interesting to implement a wide approach using different types of stabilizer, classified as disaccharides (Suc, Tre), cyclic oligosaccharide (HP-β-CD), polysaccharide (Inu) and polyol

160

(Sor) [222]. Stabilizers are able to form hydrogen bonds with proteins, which leads to water replacement. Moreover, they are able to form a matrix around the protein to reduce or prevent its mobility. This well-known effect is called "vitrification theory" [155].

The effect of the addition of stabilizers on the stability of the loaded mAb was investigated using three different mAb:stabilizer ratios (1.5:1, 2.0:1 and 2.5:1) (Table 17). It has previously been described that a mAb:stabilizer ratio of 2.0:1 increased the stability of mAb during a spray-drying process [218]. In our study, higher and lower ratios were also investigated to evaluate their influence on the stability of our own mAb, which was stressed by heat successively through HME and 3DP.

The yield of the SD process, when such biotherapeutic is involved, was expected to be ranged between 70% and 50% (w/w) in the worst case [161]. Surprisingly, it was observed that the yields were very high and even higher than 100%, especially when HP-β-CD was used as stabilizer (Table 17). Indeed, formulations SD_13, SD_14, SD_15 were characterized by a yield of 103.5%, 106.1% and 100.8%, respectively (n=1). Moreover, the yields observed from formulations SD_10, SD_11 and SD_12 were 93.1%, 102.8% and 99.1%, respectively. It seemed that similar trends were obtained when inulin was added as stabilizer (Table 17). This may be related to the fact that cyclodextrins and inulin are able to form aggregates as soon as their concentrations are higher than the critical aggregation concentration [223,224].

Inulin also promotes gel formation, which increases the viscosity of the solution [225,226]. The increase in the viscosity could influence the BE process by altering the ultrafiltration capacity of the system. Therefore, the filtration that is performed after the BE step may retain potential aggregates of carbohydrate, which may lead to a decrease in the concentration of the mAb or an alteration of the mAb:stabilizer ratio. The latter point could appear if self-assembled carbohydrates aggregates are soluble.

The yield of the other formulations (Tre, Suc, Sor) ranged between 74.5% and 89.8% (Table 17). These results were higher than those previously described in the literature (between 50% and 70% (w/w)) [227]. Therefore, the selected parameters based on our in-house protocol seemed adapted to the process and to the selected compounds.

The mAb formulation was performed using BE and no instabilities were found between the initial mAb reference solution (provided by UCB Pharma) and the BE step. The percentage of HMWS after BE was similar to that observed from the mAb reference solution (2.6 ± 0.4%) (Table 18).

After SD, there was no significant formation of HMWS for mAb:stabilizer ratios of 1.5:1 and 2.0:1, regardless of the nature of the stabilizer (p-value > 0.05) (Table 18). In contrast, when a ratio of 2.5:1 was used, the percentage of HMWS was increased after the SD process, regardless of the nature of the stabilizers, except for Suc and Tre (p-value > 0.05) (Table 18). Indeed, disaccharides such as Suc and Tre may create a more viscous glassy matrix to protect protein molecules [228,229]. Following these results, the 2.5:1 ratio was discarded. Moreover, as ratios of 1.5:1 and 2.0:1 showed similar results, the 2.0:1 ratio was selected for further investigations as it allowed a higher proportion of mAb versus stabilizers (Table 18). Consequently, a higher amount of powder in the 1.5:1 ratio should be used in comparison with powder in the 2.0:1 ratio to include the same amount of mAb. This higher amount would lead to a more difficult handling of the powder during the HME process. However, both ratios were used to produce 3DP implants and were characterized to ensure the study consistency.

The LMWS level was also assessed and no fragmentation was observed on raw mAb. A similar observation was made after BE and SD, regardless of the mAb:stabilizer ratio (Table 18).

Table 18. Comparison of HMWS and LMWS levels of mAb formulation (mAb:stabilizer ratios: 1.5:1; 2.0:1 and 2.5:1) after BE (n=1), SD and HME (n = 3, mean ± SD). The monomer content as well as the HMWS and LMWS levels of the mAb reference are shown.

| mAb:stab. ratio | | 1.5:1 | | | 2.0:1 | | | 2.5:1 | | |
Process Stab.		BE	SD	HME	BE	SD	HME	BE	SD	HME
SUC	HMWS (%)	2.5	2.7 ± 0.3	3.2 ± 0.2	2.5	2.8 ± 0.1	3.3 ± 0.3	2.9	3.51 ± 0.04	4.2 ± 0.2
	LMWS (%)	ND	ND	ND	ND	ND	ND	ND	ND	ND
TRE	HMWS (%)	2.5	2.8 ± 0.8	3.2 ± 0.5	2.8	3.2 ± 0.5	3.8 ± 0.5	2.9	3.54 ± 0.02	4.3 ± 0.1
	LMWS (%)	ND	ND	ND	ND	ND	ND	ND	ND	ND
SOR	HMWS (%)	2.3	3.1 ± 0.1	14.6 ± 0.5	2.5	3.3 ± 0.2	11.2 ± 0.4	2.4	3.22 ± 0.03	8.9 ± 0.3
	LMWS (%)	ND	ND	ND	ND	ND	0.4 ± 0.1	ND	0.00 ± 0.01	0.2 ± 0.1
INU	HMWS (%)	2.5	3.7 ± 0.2	5.4 ± 0.2	2.5	3.6 ± 0.3	4.9 ± 0.1	2.6	4.05 ± 0.02	4.8 ± 0.1
	LMWS (%)	ND	ND	ND	ND	ND	ND	ND	ND	ND
HP-β-CD	HMWS (%)	2.8	3.0 ± 0.3	9.4 ± 0.8	2.5	3.5 ± 0.5	6.3 ± 0.2	2.8	4.10 ± 0.02	8.0 ± 0.5
	LMWS (%)	ND	ND	ND	ND	ND	0.10 ± 0.05	ND	0.02 ± 0.01	0.23 ± 0.02
mAb reference solution	Monomer (%)	97.4 ± 0.4								
	HMWS (%)	2.6 ± 0.4								
	LMWS (%)	ND								

*(Stab.: stabilizer, ND: not detected)

II.3 Extrusion of mAb-loaded printable filaments

All filaments were successfully prepared (Process-11, Thermo Fisher Scientific, USA), with a diameter between 1.70 and 1.75 mm as recommended to feed the FDM 3D printer (as described in 'Materials and methods' – section II.2.2) [71].

At the beginning of the study, several trials were performed using a mAb loading of 20% (w/w) in the filaments. Using this percentage, a high amount of mAb was required and it was observed that such high loading tended to increase the burst effect due to percolation issues. This effect occurred as the PLGA matrix was not able to sustain the release of the loaded mAb within the first hours of dissolution [103,130]. Therefore, the loading percentage was progressively decreased. It was shown that the maximal percentage that allowed minimal degradation of the mAb, optimal homogeneity within the filament and minimal burst effect from the 3DP devices was a loading of 15% (w/w). Interestingly, using a theoretical loading of 15% (w/w) led to a higher yield than that observed from a loading of 20% (w/w), regardless of the type of stabilizer and the ratios (65 ± 4% vs 44 ± 6%) (Table 17).

Afterwards, the mAb-loaded spray-dried powder was mixed with PLGA and PEG and extruded to make printable filaments. It was shown that the percentage of HMWS was increased due to the use of relatively high temperatures, regardless of the nature of the stabilizer (p-value < 0.0001) (Table 18).

However, it was demonstrated that the percentage of HMWS reached 6.4 ± 0.2%, 11.2 ± 0.5% and 4.9 ± 0.1% when HP-β-CD (HME_14), Sor (HME_8) and Inu (HME_11) were added to the formulations (mAb:stabilizer ratio 2.0:1) (Fig. 67). In contrast, Suc and Tre seemed the most adapted to stabilizing the mAb during the HME process, which was performed at 90 °C. Indeed, the percentages of HMWS increased to only 3.3 ± 0.3% (Suc, HME_2) and 3.8 ± 0.5% (Tre, HME_5), respectively (Fig. 67). No significant difference was highlighted for both disaccharides after HME (p-value > 0.05).

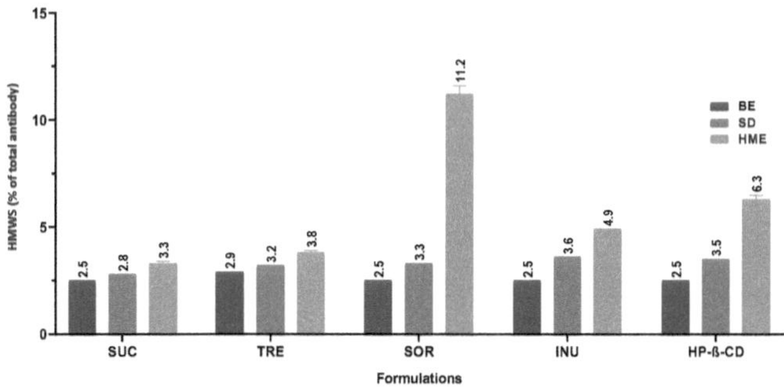

Fig. 67. Comparison of the HMWS levels for the mAb formulation (mAb:stabilizer ratio 2.0:1) containing Suc, Tre, HP-β-CD, Sor and Inu after BE, SD and HME (n=3, mean ± SD).

*Formulations are summarized as SUC: SD_2 (BE, SD), HME_2 (HME); TRE: SD_5 (BE, SD), HME_5 (HME); SOR: SD_8 (BE, SD), HME_8 (HME); INU: SD_11 (BE, SD), HME_11 (HME); HP-β-CD: SD_14 (BE, SD), HME_14 (HME) (Table 17).

In addition, the percentage of LMWS was evaluated after HME. It was observed that fragmentation appeared when HP-β-CD and Sor were added to the formulations (Table 18). In contrast, no LMWS were shown with Suc, Tre and Inu (Table 18). The fragmentation was induced when high temperatures were used. Indeed, non-enzymatic reactions could lead to the fragmentation of disulphide or peptide bonds, specifically in the hinge region. Furthermore, high temperatures can promote deamidation of amino acids such as asparagine and glutamine. This phenomenon is accelerated at acidic pH [140,230].

Nevertheless, these results showed that a higher HMWS level was observed when the formulation contained Sor (Fig. 67). It could be due to the inability of Sor to promote mAb stability during transfer of heat. In the literature, Sor was used to stabilize mAb in solution or during a freeze-drying process. However, aggregation was promoted due to the recrystallization of Sor during storage [168,229]. Crystallization may lead to a loss of protein-stabilizer interactions [155]. There could be a similar effect during HME, where enough energy was provided to Sor to recrystallize and thus promote the degradation of the mAb. This hypothesis may be confirmed using x-ray diffraction identification to assess the crystallinity of the Sor in further experiment.

HP-β-CD and Inu were less effective at maintaining mAb stability during HME in comparison to the other stabilizers (Suc and Tre). HP-β-CD has been reported to interact with proteins via the hydroxypropyl functions [231]. Instabilities could be due to the lack of interactions between mAb and cyclodextrin. Inu is a polysaccharide with a higher Mw, where steric hindrance and reduced flexibility may lead to reduced interactions between Inu and mAb [165]. According to the evaluation of HMWS and LMWS levels, the mAb integrity was ensured during HME using Tre and Suc as stabilizers (Table 18).

Overall, Suc and Tre seemed to be the most suitable stabilizers for stabilizing the formulations over the successive production steps. Interestingly, both compounds are characterized by similar structures, which belong to disaccharide class. It has already been noted that such derivatives are able to create hydrogen bonds with the protein. They also form a glassy matrix to avoid protein-protein interactions, which are known to promote aggregation issues [155,221,228,232,233]. Furthermore, these two disaccharides were characterized by a high T_g around 120 °C and 60 °C for Tre and Suc, respectively. The stabilizing effect of these compounds is influenced by their ability to stay in amorphous state and promote the vitrification effect [165].

In addition, to be more consistent, printable filaments were also produced using the ratios 1.5:1 and 2.5:1 (Table 18). Interestingly, depending on the stabilizer, these ratios were characterized by similar or even higher HMWS than the 2.0:1 ratio. For instance, HP-β-CD showed a higher proportion of HMWS for the ratios 1.5:1 (9.4 ± 0.8%) and 2.5:1 (8.0 ± 0.5%), in comparison with the ratio 2.0:1 (3.5 ± 0.5%) (Table 18). This last observation supported the selection of the 2.0:1 ratio after the SD step.

Finally, the mAb loading was assessed on the printable filaments (with a loading of 15% (w/w)) before the printing process. This showed that the loadings of all the filaments were similar to the theoretical loading (15% w/w), with very low standard deviations (Table 19). These results indicated that the manufacturing process was suitable and reproducible to produce uniform printable filaments with homogeneous dispersion of mAb.

II.4   3DP of the mAb delivery devices

Slicing software (ThinkerCAD™, Autodesk®, USA) was used to design a model of a 3DP DDS with a cylindrical shape that could be implantable (as described in 'Materials and methods' – section II.3.3). As 3DP is a relatively new process in the pharmaceutical field, techniques such as HME and electrospinning have been widely investigated to produce cylindrical implants [102,128,129]. Indeed, HME is able to produce rod (cylindrical)- or film-based shapes depending on the shape of the die. In the literature, 3DP implants have been designed using the Etonogestrel implant developed by Merck as a reference. The development of the cylindrical DDS was characterized by a diameter of 2 mm and a length of 40 mm [55]. The 3DP allows the production of devices in a layer-wise manner with a high control of the deposition (e.g. height of the layers). Furthermore, FDM technology is performed to build devices with no post-processing step [42].

The printing process was performed at 20 °C (environmental condition). The physical state of the filaments could be quickly modified due to the temperature as their T_g was around 21 °C. Therefore, at 20 °C, filaments were able to be printed as their stiffness was preserved. However, the handling of the filaments induced heat transfer by conduction. This phenomenon was greater when the filaments were loaded in the print head. Indeed, they were too soft to travel along the feeding gears [234]. To limit these issues, 3DP had to be performed using a "flexible hot flow"

MKE-250 modular printing head (Hyrel®, USA) (as described in 'Materials and methods' – section II.3.3).

The DDS resolution was macroscopically evaluated and, when the infill was set at 100%, a fully solid DDS was expected (Fig. 68). The resolution was the fidelity between the initial CAD files (design) and the 3DP devices, which depends on the FDM technique and printed material (Fig. 68a) [235]. Immediate visualization showed defects and a lack of matter at the top of the devices (Fig. 68b). The Hyrel® 30M 3D printer (Hyrel®, USA) works with a fixed print head and a mobile build platform (as described in 'Materials and methods' – section II.3.3). The hypothesis was that the platform motion represented the limitation of the process, especially when small pieces were built. The printing step was performed with a deposition rate of 1 mm/s for the first layer and of 10 mm/s for the following layers to improve the resolution of the DDS.

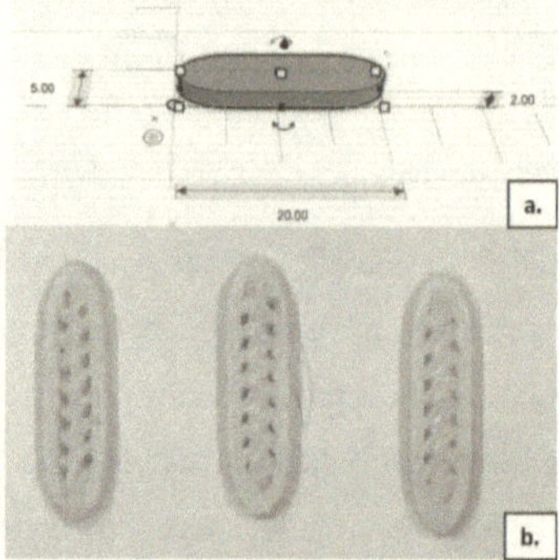

Fig. 68. (**a.**) Implantable device (20 x 5 x 2 mm (L x W x H)) designed with TinkerCad™, (**b.**) 3D-printed devices (100% (w/w)) obtained using the Hyrel® 30 M system 3DP.

Extraction of mAb was performed on 3DP DDS to evaluate the percentage of both HMWS and LMWS. As mentioned above, Suc and Tre were able to stabilize the mAb during the SD and HME processes. 3DP was performed at 105 °C. This deposition temperature allowed the adhesion of the first layer to the build platform as well as between the layers themselves. Layer thicknesses of 0.1 mm and 0.3 mm were evaluated. However, it may be interesting to mention that 3DP devices were printed using all the previously mentioned stabilizers (i.e. Tre, Suc, HP-β-CD, Inu and Sor) at all ratios (1.5:1, 2.0:1 and 2.5:1). As expected, it was observed that a higher degradation was observed with the 2.5:1 ratio. Moreover, similar results were retrieved between the 1.5:1 and 2.0:1 ratios. This last observation was consistent with our previous selection of the 2.0:1 (Fig. 69).

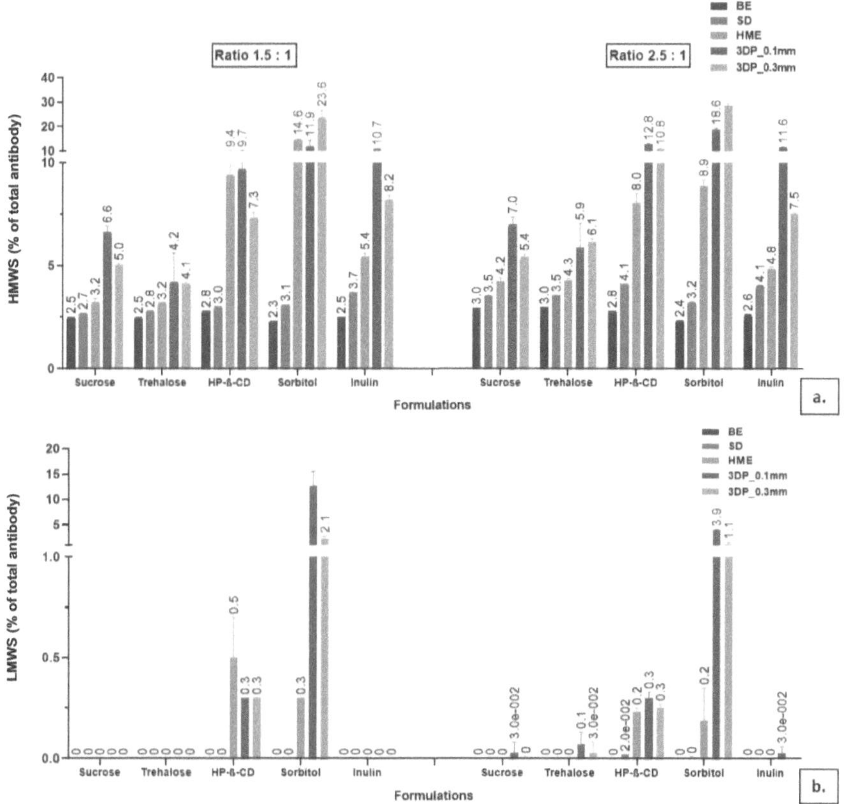

Fig. 69. Comparison of the HMWS (**a.**) and LMWS (**b.**) levels for the mAb formulations at ratios 1.5:1 and 2.5:1 containing Suc, Tre, HP-β-CD, Sor and Inu after BE, SD, HME and 3DP (n=3, mean ± SD).

*Formulations are summarized as SUC: SD_1 (BE, SD), HME_1 (HME), 3DP_1 (3DP_0.1 mm) and 3DP_2 (3DP_0.3 mm); TRE: SD_4 (BE, SD), HME_4 (HME), 3DP_7 (3DP_0.1 mm) and 3DP_8 (3DP_0.3 mm); HP-β-CD: SD_13 (BE, SD), HME_13 (HME) and 3DP_25 (3DP_0.1 mm) and 3DP_26 (3DP_0.3 mm); SOR: SD_7 (BE, SD), HME_7 (HME) and 3DP_13 (3DP_0.1 mm) and 3DP_14 (3DP_0.3 mm); INU: SD_10 (BE, SD), HME_10 (HME) and 3DP_19 (3DP_0.1 mm) and 3DP_20 (3DP_0.3 mm) at the ratio 1.5:1; and SUC: SD_3 (BE, SD), HME_3 (HME), 3DP_5 (3DP_0.1 mm) and 3DP_6 (3DP_0.3 mm); TRE: SD_6 (BE, SD), HME_6 (HME), 3DP_11 (3DP_0.1 mm) and 3DP_12 (3DP_0.3 mm); HP-β-CD: SD_15 (BE, SD), HME_15 (HME) and 3DP_29 (3DP_0.1 mm) and 3DP_30 (3DP_0.3 mm); SOR: SD_9 (BE, SD), HME_9 (HME) and 3DP_17 (3DP_0.1 mm) and 3DP_18 (3DP_0.3 mm); INU: SD_12 (BE, SD), HME_12 (HME) and 3DP_23 (3DP_0.1 mm) and 3DP_24 (3DP_0.3 mm) at the ratio 2.5:1 (Table 17).

Compared to the level observed after HME, the percentage of HMWS increased after 3DP, regardless of the layer height or the nature of the disaccharide (Fig. 70). However, the HMWS levels were significantly higher when a layer thickness of 0.1 mm was used (p-value < 0.0001 and p-value < 0.001, respectively). For instance, the HMWS percentage increased from 3.3 ± 0.1% (HME_16) and 3.8 ± 0.1% (HME_18) after HME to 4.7 ± 0.3% (3DP_34) and 4.8 ± 0.1% (3DP_41) after 3DP, with a layer thickness of 0.3 mm, when Suc and Tre were used, respectively (Fig. 70). This was attributed to the relatively high temperature during 3DP. Furthermore, as previously observed, a layer thickness of 0.1 mm is more damaging than one of 0.3 mm (Fig. 70). This may be explained by the extended area of contact between the nozzle of the printer and the printed devices at 0.1 mm of layer thickness (as previously described in the part I).

Despite the addition of Suc or Tre, it was demonstrated that a significant increase in HMWS appeared after 3DP. Therefore, it was hypothesized that the addition of a hydrophobic amino acid such as Leu could enhance the stability of the loaded mAb. Both disaccharides have already been investigated with Leu to improve the mAb powder properties during the SD process. Combinations of stabilizers and Leu (5% (w/w)) have already been investigated and showed promising results on powder characteristics (e.g. powder dispersion) [236].

To improve the amorphous glassy state of the powder, a mixture of selected disaccharides (Suc and Tre) and Leu was evaluated. It seemed interesting to promote this glassy state as it was expected to improve the stability of mAb. Indeed, Tre and Leu-based formulations have already been described as ensuring good protein stabilization by promoting this glassy state [237,238]. Therefore, 3DP devices loaded with Suc-Leu and Tre-Leu were printed using a layer thickness of 0.3 mm.

To evaluate the potential benefit of the addition of Leu on the stability of the loaded mAb, HMWS levels were evaluated after each process (from SD to 3DP). After 3DP, these levels were 4.4 ± 0.2% and 3.6 ± 0.1% for 3DP_37 (Suc-Leu) and 3DP_44 (Tre-Leu), respectively (Fig. 70). These levels were compared to those obtained when Suc and Tre were used alone. It was demonstrated that the addition of Leu to Suc and Tre decreased the production of HMWS. However, the decrease in HMWS was significant only with the association of Tre-Leu (p-value < 0.0001).

The rate of increase was compared as a ratio over the whole process (between 3DP and SD). Indeed, following the addition of Leu to Tre, the percentage of HMWS increased by about 16% versus 50% when Tre was formulated alone (Fig. 70). The same trend was observed when Leu was added to Suc, with higher HMWS levels (Suc-Leu: 33% vs Suc: 68% increase) (Fig. 70).

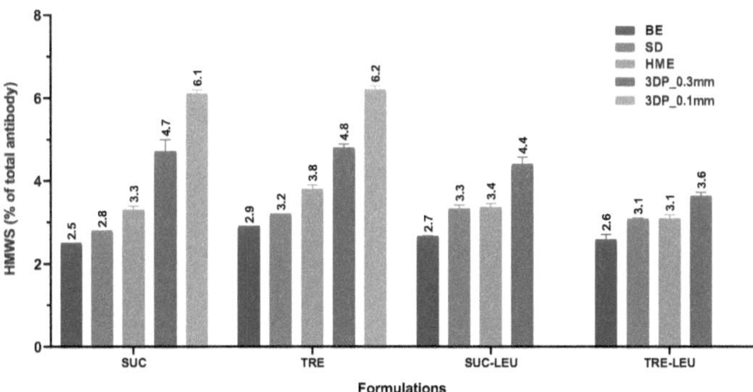

Fig. 70. Comparison of the HMWS levels for the mAb formulation (mAb:stabilizer ratio 2.0:1) containing Suc, Tre, Suc-Leu and Tre-Leu after BE, SD, HME and 3DP (n=3, mean ± SD).

*Formulations are summarized as SUC: SD_16 (BE, SD), HME_16 (HME), 3DP_34 (3DP_0.3 mm) and 3DP_31 (3DP_0.1 mm); TRE: SD_18 (BE, SD), HME_18 (HME), 3DP_41 (3DP_0.3 mm) and 3DP_37 (3DP_0.1 mm); SUC-LEU: SD_17 (BE, SD), HME_17 (HME) and 3DP_37 (3DP_0.3 mm); TRE-LEU: SD_19 (BE, SD), HME_19 (HME) and 3DP_44 (3DP_0.3 mm) (Table 17).

LMWS levels after 3DP were also evaluated. A slight increase in LMWS (around 0.05 ± 0.04%) was demonstrated, regardless of the addition of Leu to Suc or Tre (data not shown).

Finally, drug loadings were assessed on 3DP DDS. The BCA results showed loadings close to the theoretical loading of 15% (w/w) (Table 19). These results were consistent with the loading of printable filaments. Thus, results were in phase with the previous observation of the uniform dispersion of mAb in the polymeric matrix expressed after HME (as previously described in experimental part III - section II.3).

Table 19. mAb loading in printable filaments and 3DP devices obtained by BCA assay (Table 17).

HME batch name	mAb loading (% w/w)	3DP batch name	mAb loading (% w/w)
HME_16	16.0 ± 0.1	3DP_34	15.8 ± 0.2
HME_17	15.2 ± 0.1	3DP_37	15.1 ± 0.2
HME_18	16.2 ± 0.1	3DP_41	16.2 ± 0.3
HME_19	15.6 ± 0.2	3DP_44	15.5 ± 0.2
HME_20	15.9 ± 0.5	3DP_45	15.5 ± 0.5

To the best of our knowledge, there is no report of this manufacturing process, which uses mAb-loaded spray-dried particles to extrude printable filaments by HME for use in FDM to create 3DP DDS. In accordance with the previous results, the increase in HMWS was directly related to the thermal degradation occurring at 90 °C and 105 °C with HME and 3DP, respectively. However, it was shown that the formulation containing Tre-Leu was able to minimize the production of HMWS and to promote mAb stability. Therefore, this formulation was investigated through *in vitro* evaluations such as dissolution tests as well as the binding capacity evaluation. Indeed, the integrity of the mAb after its release from the DDS must be preserved.

II.5 Dissolution tests

It was previously demonstrated and described that PLGA-based DDS (e.g. microparticles and implants) are characterized by triphasic release profiles. These phases include an initial burst effect (I), a latent phase with diffusion-driven release (II) and a sustained release of the drug due to the erosion of the polymer (III) [109,128,172]. To ensure a steady and sustained release of the loaded mAb over time, melt processing such as 3DP seemed adequate. To our knowledge, systems such as microparticles have shown high burst effects [170,172]. This issue could be decreased using DDS with a dense polymer matrix and larger size than the latter microparticles.

The instability of a mAb increases in liquid state and may lead to chemical degradations [158]. Moreover, it could be interesting to promote a release profile where a limited latent phase occurs. Indeed, the latent phase could lead to mAb degradation due to its retention in the polymer matrix and the medium uptake. Moreover, a linear release profile which could tend towards a "zero order kinetic" should allow a constant drug release of the mAb in the dissolution medium.

II.5.1 Optimization of the dissolution tests

II.5.1.1 Influence of the stabilizers

Dissolution tests were performed on devices from 3DP_32 to 3DP_44, which corresponded to Suc-based formulations (3DP_32/33/34), Suc-Leu-based formulations (3DP_35/36/37), Tre-based formulations (3DP_39/40/41) and Tre-Leu-based formulations (3DP_42/43/44), to evaluate the release of the loaded mAb from the corresponded DDS (Table 17). The dissolution profiles of the loaded mAb from the 3DP DDS were evaluated using 10, 50 and 100% of infill to investigate the potential influence of their microarchitecture. The weight of the devices were evaluated before the dissolution test (Table 20). These increased with the infill percentage. According to the results, 3DP devices were considered repeatable. Further investigations should focus on the repeatability of the printing and on the accuracy of the physical dimension to assess the production capability and suitability of the printer.

Table 20. Weighing of the 3DP devices used for the dissolution test.

3D batch number	Weight (mg)
3DP_32	173.9 ± 5.3
3DP_33	180.1 ± 6.7
3DP_34	202.8 ± 7.5
3DP_35	175.9 ± 6.7
3DP_36	185.2 ± 5.0
3DP_37	199.5 ± 4.2
3DP_39	181.6 ± 2.3
3DP_40	189.1 ± 2.8
3DP_41	199.4 ± 13.1
3DP_42	183.4 ± 2.7
3DP_43	191.3 ± 5.5
3DP_44	196.6 ± 3.5
3DP_45	207.8 ± 3.3

Suc-based formulations were characterized by a low burst effect. For instance, the highest value reached only 2.7 ± 0.4% within 24h from batch 3DP_35 (Fig. 71). In our study, after 6 weeks of dissolution, the percentage of release of the loaded-mAb was 18.8 ± 4.9% and 18.6 ± 4.8% from batches 3DP_32 and 3DP_33, respectively. In contrast, batch 3DP_34 only released 11.1 ± 1.4% of mAb within 6 weeks. Moreover, the percentages of release of the mAb from batch 3DP_34 were lower than those observed from both 3DP_32 and 3DP_33, regardless of the time points. Such trend could be due to the infill of 100%, which sustained the diffusion of the medium through the 3DP DDS due to the reduced contact surface that it afforded. Moreover, a lag time was observed for 4 weeks before a slight increase in the release which was then followed by a sustained release of the loaded mAb, as previously described. It was also observed that a slightly higher release was reached from a combination of Suc and Leu when compared to the Suc-based formulations (3DP_32, 3DP_33, 3DP_34). A percentage of release of 26.8 ± 4.7% was obtained from batch 3DP_36 within 6 weeks. Moreover, after 6 weeks of dissolution, the percentage of release of the loaded mAb was similar regardless of the infill percentage of the 3D DDS. Overall results showed that Suc-based formulations had a slower release than that observed from a combination of Suc and Leu. Nonetheless, no statistically significant difference was observed between the 3DP devices with Suc and Suc-Leu based formulations (f2 > 50), regardless of the infill percentage. The amount of Leu that was added in the formulation seemed to not be able to reduce the release of the loaded mAb.

Such low burst effect was already observed from PLGA-based formulations obtained by HME due to the monolithic (dense) matrix and the limited access of dissolution medium to extract the mAb [102]. For instance, Cossé et al. reported a burst release after 24h of 3.7 ± 0.2% from BSA-loaded PLGA implants produced by HME [129].

After the burst release, a phase of slow release usually appeared for 4 weeks, which corresponds to a "lag phase". This is due to the struggle of medium to penetrate into the polymer matrix and is known to be "low" during the first weeks [103,129].

However, 3DP devices with an infill of 10% (3DP_32) and 50% (3DP_33) were characterized by similar release profiles (f2 > 50). Therefore, no influence of the infill percentage was observed within 6 weeks of dissolution. This may be due to the medium uptake in the dense PLGA matrix, which decreased the mAb-diffusion process. Moreover, it was previously described in literature that only a small volume of medium was able to diffuse through the matrix during the first weeks. Even if the polymer degradation was out of the scope of this preliminary study, in the next section it is described how the polymer structure evolved over time. Indeed, the diffusion of the medium through the polymeric matrix is needed to trigger the hydrolysis and promote the erosion of the DDS [129]. Moreover, the diffusion of the medium seems to be one part of the process because a sufficient amount of water is needed to promote the dissolution of the mAb that is initially trapped in the matrix. This could explain why only a small amount of mAb was released within 6 weeks. Once the polymer was hydrated, its chemical structure was modified, which could lead to a reduction in the influence of the infill on the release of the loaded mAb. Indeed, it was demonstrated that PLGA swelling could modify the porous structure of DDS and delay the drug release as a consequence [103].

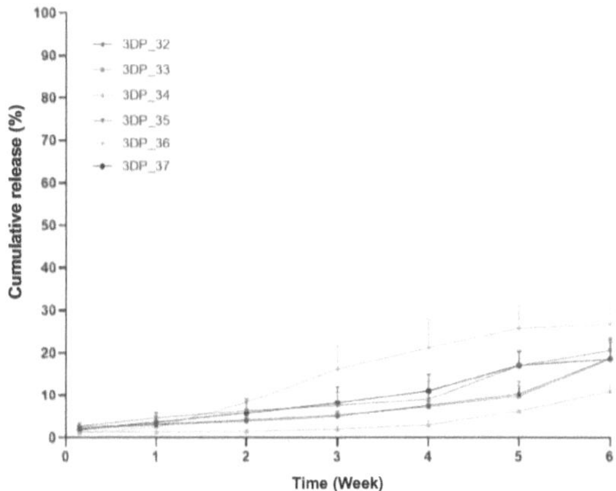

Fig. 71. In vitro release profiles of 3DP devices with different infill percentages, containing mAb stabilized with Suc (3DP_32 (10%), 3DP_33 (50%), 3DP_34 (100%)) and Suc-Leu association (3DP_35 (10%), 3DP_36 (50%), 3DP_37 (100%)) (n=3, mean ± SD). Devices were printed with a layer thickness of 0.3 mm.

Tre-based formulations showed different patterns but statistically similar types of release profiles (similarity factor (f2)) within 6 weeks from those observed with Suc-based formulations (Fig. 72). Indeed, the release of mAb from Tre-based formulations was not characterized by a lag phase during the first 4 weeks (Fig. 72). The dissolution and the subsequent diffusion of the mAb seemed to promote the release of the biotherapeutic. However, the percentage of release after 24h was not higher than 10%, regardless of the nature of the carbohydrate derivative. Formulations containing Tre, without amino acid, were characterized by a significant lower percentage of release after 6 weeks (f2 < 50). For instance, a maximal value of 33.1 ± 5.4% and 33.8 ± 2.2% was obtained from batches 3DP_39 and 3DP_41, respectively. Interestingly, batch 3DP_40 showed a different type of release profile, with a lag time for the first couple of weeks before an increase in the release to reach only 17.5 ± 2.1% within 6 weeks. The cumulative release seemed to increase after a month of dissolution, probably due to the degradation of the polymer and the higher quantity of protein available to the dissolution medium. Interestingly, different release profiles were obtained when Leu was associated to Tre in the formulation. Indeed, the percentages of release were higher over time than those observed without the addition of the amino acid. The burst effect reached 6.0 ± 2.4%, 3.3 ± 0.1% and 6.1 ± 0.5% for batches 3DP_44 (infill 100%), 3DP_43 (infill 50%) and 3DP_42 (infill 10%), respectively. After 1 week, the percentage of release of the mAb reached about 24% w/w. Then, its release from batches 3DP_44 and 3DP_43 was similar until week 6 (f2 > 50), with a cumulative release of 63.2 ± 4.7% and 62.3 ± 5.1%, respectively. The value of 3DP_42 after week 6 reached 59.4 ± 3.5%. Overall, the release of the mAb after 6 weeks when formulated with Tre was higher than observed with Suc. Tre may preserve the mAb stability in the polymeric matrix and avoid the formation of insoluble aggregates.

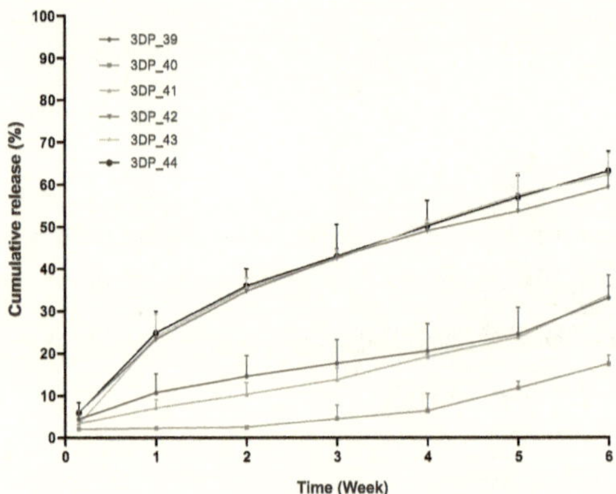

Fig. 72. In vitro release profiles of 3DP devices with different infill percentages, containing mAb stabilized with Tre (3DP_39 (10%), 3DP_40 (50%), 3DP_41 (100%)) and Tre-Leu association (3DP_42 (10%), 3DP_43 (50%), 3DP_44 (100%)) (n=3, mean ± SD). Devices were printed with a layer thickness of 0.3 mm.

In contrast, the release of the mAb was promoted by porogen-like effect or by plasticizing effect related to the tensioactive properties of Leu. This effect could be due to the ability of Leu to produce fine mAb powder particles and promote a better dispersion of them into the polymer matrix. Leu was mainly used for its property to improve the SD process and promote fine particles [167]. These particles could be quickly dissolved, leading to a higher release over time. Moreover, the addition of Leu could reduce polymer and mAb-particle interaction and therefore promote the release of the mAb.

II.5.1.2 Influence of the pH

The potential evolution of the pH in the dissolution medium was also evaluated (Fig. 73). Indeed, it has already been widely reported that the hydrolysis of PLGA acidifies the medium due to the release of both PLA and PGA residues. Such acidification tends to induce an autocatalyze, which accelerates the hydrolysis of PLGA [239]. Therefore, the release of the loaded drug would be accelerated. As already mentioned, the selected PLGA derivative, Resomer® RG 502, is characterized by a degradation time lower than 3 months [240].

Although the pH of the medium was around 7.0 within the first month of dissolution, it sharply decreased between the 5th and the 6th week (Fig. 73b). As can be seen, the lowest pH values were 4.0 ± 0.1 (3DP_39), 3.7 ± 0.2 (3DP_40) and 4.0 ± 0.1 (3DP_41) after 6 weeks of dissolution for Tre-based formulations. When Leu was added, the pH decreased from 7.0 to 4.7 ± 0.6 (3DP_42), 4.1 ± 0.1 (3DP_43) and 4.1 ± 0.1 (3DP_44) (Fig. 73b). After 6 weeks of dissolution, Suc-based formulations showed similar decrease in the pH of the medium, regardless of the addition of Leu. For instance, the pH of the medium decreased to 3.5 ± 0.1 with 3DP_34 and 3DP_37 (Suc-leu) (Fig. 73a). The highest pH value was obtained with batches 3DP_33 (4.7 ± 0.6) and 3DP_32 (4.4 ± 0.1), which contained only Suc in the formulations (Fig. 73a). The decrease in the pH could impair the integrity of the protein in the DDS. Indeed, it has previously been demonstrated that a microenvironmental pH within the PLGA structure led to the degradation of the loaded peptide [149,241].

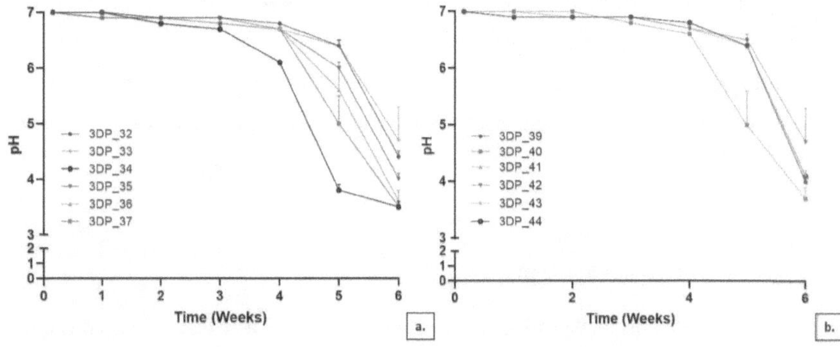

Fig. 73. *In vitro* pH variation over dissolution time of (**a.**) Suc (3DP_32/33/34) and Suc-Leu (3DP_35/36/37) and (**b.**) Tre (3DP_39/40/41) and Tre-Leu (3DP_42/43/44) based formulations (n=3, mean ± SD).

II.5.1.3 Evaluation of mAb stability

The mAb stability was also assessed during the dissolution test. The integrity of the mAb was evaluated after its release in the dissolution medium using protein monomers, as well as the LMWS and HMWS levels (Fig. 74). It was shown that a decrease in the monomer percentage was associated with an increase in either HMWS or LMWS species. Indeed, the aggregation and the fragmentation of the mAb occurring on the mAb degrades the monomer structure that is the functional Y-shaped structure of the immunoglobulin.

The highest percentages of LMWS species were obtained after 6 weeks, regardless of the type of stabilizer (Fig. 74a). In comparison with the Suc-based formulations, Tre-based formulations seemed to avoid fragmentation to a greater extent (Fig. 74a, d). Indeed, the maximal percentage of LMWS was 13.7 ± 4.6% from batch 3DP_37 (Suc-Leu) after 6 weeks of dissolution (Fig. 74a). This percentage was unexpected considering that, after 4 weeks, this level was only 0.51 ± 0.03%. The erosion of PLGA could have promoted the diffusion of mAb from the matrix core. During the erosion step, which occurred between week 4 and 6, acidic species were produced, leading to a decrease in the pH. This could impair the stability of the mAb. In contrast, the highest percentages of LMWS were obtained from batches 3DP_34 (3.4 ± 2.3%) and 3DP_36 (3.0 ± 1.0%), which were formulated with Suc and a Suc-Leu association, respectively. Tre-based formulations showed the highest pH value for the medium, with the highest value from 3DP_40 (1.4 ± 0.7%) after 6 weeks. The other devices were characterized by a value increase lower than 1%.

As already mentioned, the HMWS level may be correlated with that of the LMWS. Indeed, an increase in the HMWS percentage was also observed over time. The highest percentages were observed from batch 3DP_39 (9.0 ± 0.1%), where mAb was stabilized with Tre (Fig. 74e). It was observed that the highest HMWS percentages were mainly observed after 4-6 weeks of dissolution. Then, a decrease was shown for all the 3DP DDS. The hypothesis was the decrease in the pH in the dissolution medium induced the production of soluble and insoluble aggregates. Before quantification, the medium was filtered and, therefore, only soluble aggregates were considered to evaluate the HMWS level. This filtration could have lowered the amount of mAb available for its characterization by SEC. This mAb concentration can be close to the lowest standard, leading to a lower signal-to-noise ratio when compared to other standards.

This hypothesis may be confirmed as a decrease in monomer percentage was observed, regardless of the 3DP devices (Fig. 74c, f). Such decrease may be due to the degradation of mAb during the dissolution test. As previously explained, the pH of the dissolution medium decreased due to the PLGA degradation over time.

The percentage of both HMWS and monomers was assessed. Indeed, all monomer values decreased, while the lowest pH value was obtained after six weeks. Devices 3DP_36 and 3DP_37 showed large decreases in the monomer levels, which were 30.3 ± 7.0% and 31.1 ± 10.7%, respectively. These samples showed a monomer level of 91.8 ± 0.2% (3DP_36) and 92.7 ± 0.2% (3DP_37) after 4 weeks (Fig. 74c). As mentioned previously, the degradation of PLGA during its erosion generates acidic species, which lead to a drop in the pH of the medium. This drop is needed to extract the trapped mAb entity into the 3DP-device matrices. However, the pH in the PLGA matrix (microclimate pH) has been described as lower than that of the dissolution medium [241]. This deleterious environment may have led to higher mAb instabilities. It could explain the decrease in monomers that were quantified by SEC.

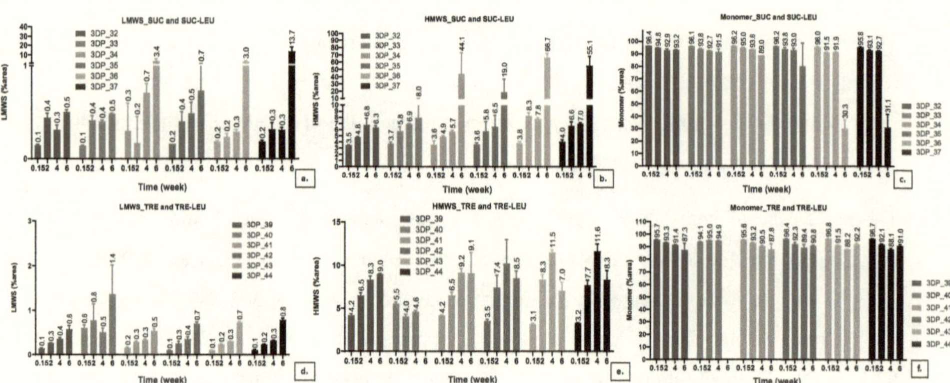

Fig. 74. Comparison of monomer, HMWS and LMWS levels of mAb Suc- (a,b,c) and Tre-based formulations (d,e,f) during in vitro dissolution tests performed on the mAb-loaded devices (n=3, mean ± SD).

178

II.5.1.4 Binding capacity of the mAb

It was also interesting to investigate the mAb binding capacity 24h after its release and compare the results to the concentration obtained by SEC at 280 nm (Fig. 75). ELISA was performed to assess the binding capacity of the mAb to its target. During this assay, the integrity of the Fab and more precisely, the complementary-determining regions were evaluated. Indeed, the binding capacity of the mAb would decrease if degradations occured on the complementary determining regions. The affinity of mAb is a key parameter to ensure its further efficacy in therapy. Suc-based formulations showed around 100% of relative binding capacity for 3DP_34 (103.3 ± 0.5%), and 3DP_33 (98.3 ± 1.5%), or less for 3DP_32, with 82.4 ± 3.6% (Fig. 75). However, the binding percentages were all higher than 100% when Leu was added to the formulation. The relative binding capacities of 3DP_35, 3DP_36 and 3DP_37 were 119.9 ± 4.8%, 124.3 ± 4.1% and 120.1 ± 2.1%, respectively. Tre-based formulations were characterized by binding capacities of 116.8 ± 4.7% (3DP_39), 121.7 ± 4.3% (3DP_40) and 117.0 ± 0.9% (3DP_41) (Fig. 75b). In contrast, when Leu was added to these formulations, the binding capacity of the mAb drastically decreased to 85.6% ± 3.7%, 92.3 ± 12.3% and 92.6 ± 3.8% from batches 3DP_42, 3DP_43 and 3DP_44, respectively.

In accordance with the results obtained after 24h, it was expected that the combination of carbohydrate and Leu would improve the mAb stability. In fact, it was shown that LMWS and HMWS levels were low and the integrity of the mAb was assumed to be preserved. Relative binding capacities are shown for all mAb samples after 24h of release.

The formulation of interest made of Tre and Leu was characterized by the lowest relative binding capacity in comparison with the other formulations. Nevertheless, this formulation was selected because of the aforementioned data and release profiles. The mAb stability when Tre-Leu association was added into the formulation showed convincing results.

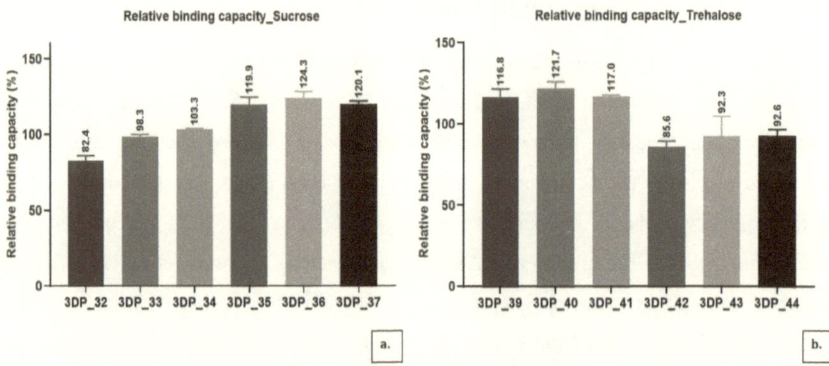

Fig. 75. Relative binding capacity of mAb release after 24h of dissolution with Suc- (a.) and Tre-based formulation devices (b.) (n=3, mean ± SD).

All these results were obtained using a volume of 1 mL of PBS following a dissolution-test protocol adapted from [242]. As the acidification of the medium was the main limitation to the mAb stability, it was interesting to avoid the pH decrease by improving the buffering capacity using a higher volume of PBS (e.g. 5 mL) during dissolution testing. Consequently, the release profiles described in the next section were assessed using Tre-Leu association (3DP_45) in a volume of 5 mL of PBS. The batch 3DP_45 was made of the same theoretical compositions and same parameters as those used to produce 3DP_42, 3DP_43 and 3DP_44 (Table 17).

II.5.2 Characterization of the release profile using optimized conditions

II.5.2.1 Release profile and PLGA degradation

The release of the mAb from 3DP_45 was characterized by a low burst release of 2.0 ± 0.3% within 24h (Fig. 76a). As mentioned previously, this was attributed to the limited access of the medium to dissolve and promote the diffusion of the loaded mAb.

As previously observed, the sustained release occurred over time, starting with a slow release phase (latent phase) within the first weeks. Indeed, between week 1 and 4, only 10.6 ± 1.9% of mAb were released (Fig. 76a). As previously explained, this was associated with the difficulty of the medium to penetrate the PLGA matrix. Water diffusion from the surface to the centre of the devices led to the swelling of PLGA [103,129]. Then, an increase in the percentage of release of the mAb was observed in the following weeks. The cumulative release accelerated and increased from $17.3 \pm 2.8\%$ after 5 weeks to $57.8 \pm 2.5\%$ after 12 weeks. Finally, a low release phase was observed to reach $59.7 \pm 2.3\%$ within 15 weeks (Fig. 76a).

The release of the mAb was dependent on the penetration of water inside the device, which allows the diffusion of the mAb through the pores of the DDS. In addition, the diffusion of the mAb from the dense PLGA matrix is also promoted with its degradation to increase this porous network [102]. Degradation/erosion of the RG502 was evaluated from the 3DP DDS during the dissolution test (Fig. 76b). PLGA was degraded by hydrolytic cleavage of its ester linkages, which produces oligomers of PLGA and leads to erosion of the device [243]. Erosion is the diffusion of oligomers (or monomers) of PLGA from the matrix to the dissolution medium. The PLGA derivative, Resomer® RG502, was characterized by an initial Mw of $17\ 867 \pm 577$ g/mol. This result was consistent with the literature [244].

Initially, the RG502 hydration occurred during the first weeks of the dissolution test. Water penetrated from the surface to the centre. Degradation of the polymer was marginally observed, and the pH value of the surrounding medium remained constant (Fig. 76). Then, its degradation increased after 3 weeks, with a loss of around 20% ($14\ 367 \pm 462$ g/mol) of the RG502 initial mass. This loss was due to the hydrolytic degradation of the RG502 in oligomers into the devices. Erosion started after 3 weeks, in accordance with the decrease in the pH of the medium (Fig. 76a). This erosion is driven by the oligomers (or monomers) generated from the RG502 matrix. During the first weeks of dissolution, mainly degradation occurred, but the onset of erosion was triggered and accelerated with the pH drop. Therefore, the autocatalysis accelerated the erosion and increased both PLGA degradation and mAb release. For instance, a loss of 64% (5373 ± 1217 g/mol) of the initial mass of the PLGA was observed after 7 weeks of dissolution (Fig. 76b). Interestingly, the pH value decreased from 7.0 to $6.3 \pm 0.1\%$, which also demonstrated the highest rate of erosion. No further degradation was observed after this main degradation and the Mw of the polymer remained stable around $6\ 000$ g/mol (Fig. 76b). Moreover, the erosion rate decreased after week 7. This statement was demonstrated by the increase in the pH value in the following weeks, from $6.7 \pm 0.1\%$ (week 8) to $7.0 \pm 0.1\%$ after 15 weeks (Fig. 76a). It was previously reported that erosion of an RG502-based 15% (w/w) BSA-loaded implant stopped after 7 weeks (50-60 days) [129]. Ghalanbor et al. demonstrated that incomplete erosion was correlated to an incomplete release of BSA [240]. Therefore, the observation made from our 3DP mAb-loaded DDP was consistent with the literature. However, the release of the mAb was promoted within 15 weeks and the pH values remained slightly acidic due to the generation of oligomers and their diffusion into the dissolution medium. This diffusion may be due to the pore formation in the matrix and constant water diffusion from the surface to the centre of the 3DP devices. Several phenomena (i.e. diffusion, erosion) occurred during the release mechanism and could evolve in phases from the surface towards the centre of the devices. No investigation on PLGA degradation longer than 10 weeks was shown in this study. Indeed, the sample generated after 10 weeks in the dissolution medium remained insoluble in chloroform. PLGA and mAb may form insoluble aggregates over time. A similar observation has been reported in the literature and was explained by the formation of thioester bonds between BSA and the PLGA matrix [130]. Furthermore, this observation was consistent with the low release phase observed after 10 weeks of dissolution and the incomplete mAb release after 15 weeks (Fig. 76a).

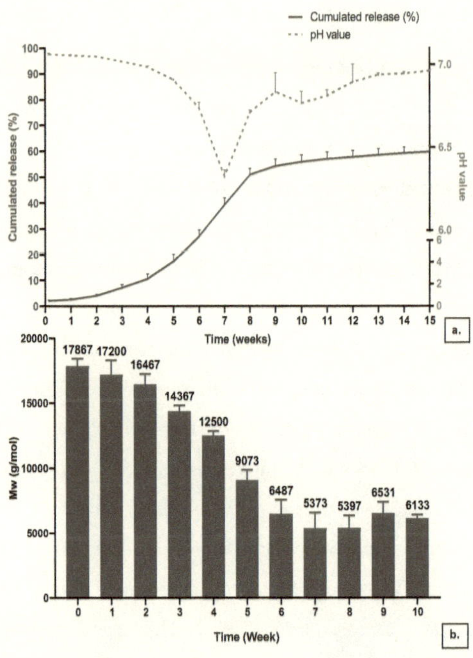

Fig. 76. (**a**) *In vitro* dissolution profiles of 3DP DDS containing mAb stabilized with Tre-Leu formulation (3DP_45) (blue solid line) and variation of pH values of the surrounding medium over dissolution time (red dashed line) (n=3, mean ± SD). (**b**) Degradation of the PLGA contained in 3DP DDS over 10 weeks in the dissolution medium at 37 °C (n=3, mean ± SD).

II.5.2.2 mAb stability and affinity over release

The sustained release of the mAb was demonstrated. However, the rehydration and the diffusion of the mAb in the dissolution medium led to mAb instabilities (Fig. 77). These instabilities were promoted by the aqueous medium and the decrease in the pH. This decrease could promote interactions between PLGA and mAb and could decrease the integrity of the mAb inside the DDS. Indeed, it has previously been demonstrated that the microenvironmental pH within a PLGA-based device led to the degradation of a loaded peptide [149,241]. Therefore, HMWS and LMWS levels, as well as the monomer content, were assessed during the dissolution test (Fig. 76a).

The highest HMWS levels generated in the dissolution medium were observed between week 6 (25.4 ± 3.6%) and week 8 (25.9 ± 3.1%) (Fig. 77). This increase was correlated with the highest erosion rate, as previously discussed, and the decrease in the pH to 6.3 ± 0.1 at week 7 (Fig. 76a). Interestingly, a slight increase in LMWS was observed (< 0.7%) during the first 9 weeks of dissolution. However, LMWS levels increased to 17.0 ± 5.7% after 10 weeks (Fig. 77). This level remained high, with a value of 15.4 ± 5.2% after 14 weeks (Fig. 77). Fragmentation was observed at a delayed stage of the dissolution test. It may be due to the hydration of the core of the PLGA-based devices, which occurred after the main erosion of the matrix. Therefore the decrease in the pH, combined with the complexity of extracting the mAb from the core, appeared more deleterious than during the main erosion process. As shown by the pH value of 6.7 ± 0.1% (week 10), acidic species continued to be extracted from the matrix (Fig. 76a).

The monomer content reached 96.5 ± 0.3% after 24h (i.e. during the burst release) (Fig. 77). This showed a decrease of monomer in the dissolution medium over time due to the instabilities during the dissolution test. The monomer content decreased to 74.1 ± 3.6% and 64.6 ± 3.3% after 6 and 12 weeks, respectively (Fig. 77).

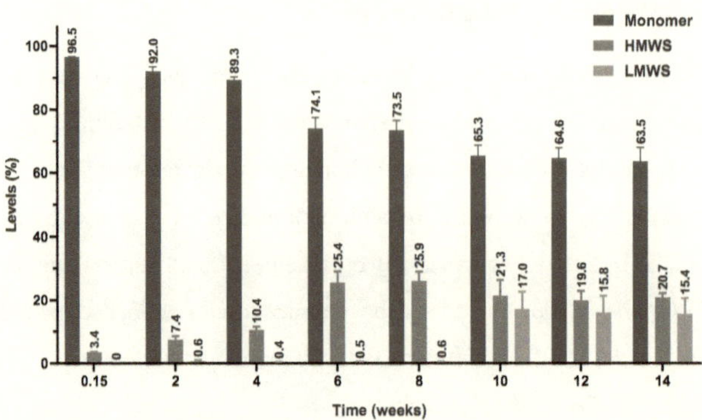

Fig. 77. Comparison of monomer, HMWS and LMWS levels (%) of the released mAb from 3DP_45 during the *in vitro* dissolution test (n=3, mean ± SD). The mAb reference solution (provided by UCB Pharma) was characterized with 97.4 ± 0.4% (monomer), 2.6 ± 0.4% (HMWS) and no LMWS.

ELISA was finally performed to evaluate the binding capacity of mAb after its diffusion from the devices to the dissolution medium. Despite the decrease in the monomer content, it seemed interesting to evaluate the mAb binding to its target.

The binding capacity of mAb was found to be 69.0 ± 1.5% after 24h (Fig. 78). This value was lower than expected from the low HMWS level and the high monomer content (96.5 ± 0.3%) previously observed (Fig. 77). Indeed, the monomer content was at its maximum after 24h of dissolution. The binding capacity after 24h could be directly associated with the degradation of mAb during the manufacturing process. A slight decrease in the binding capacity was demonstrated after 5 weeks (66.2 ± 3.8%) (Fig. 78). After 10 and 15 weeks, the binding capacity drastically decreased to 43.8 ± 6.8% and 38.8 ± 7.9%, respectively (Fig. 78). These low values may be explained by the increase in the LMWS and HMWS levels, which impaired the binding of the mAb after 10 weeks.

These results showed that complementary methods are needed to characterize the mAb integrity. Indeed, all the results previously collected and described in this study were mainly obtained by SEC, which allowed identification of HMWS and LMWS levels. Further investigations of the structure could be helpful to evaluate the degradation of the mAb and explain these lower binding capacities. For instance, it could be interesting to evaluate the secondary structure of the mAb using an analytical method such as circular dichroism. Indeed, it was reported that forced degradation at temperatures higher than 60 °C led to notable structural changes such as loss of β-sheet and unordered structures [245].

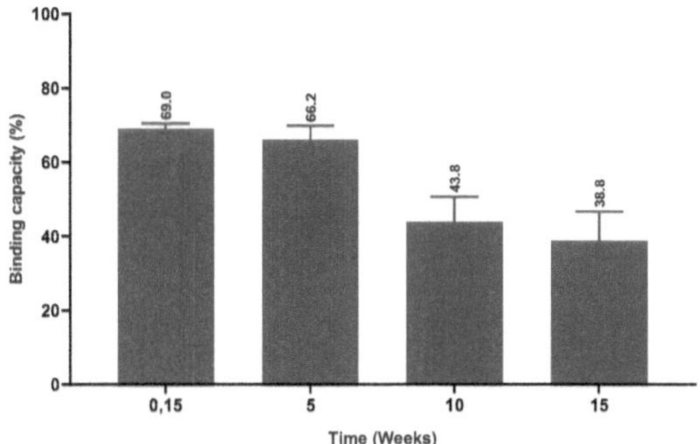

Fig. 78. Comparison of the binding capacity of the released mAb from 3DP_7 after 24h, 5, 10 and 15 weeks of dissolution (n=3, mean ± SD).

The optimization of the amount of medium in the dissolution test (5 mL) allowed characterizing and following the release of the mAb over 15 weeks, which was not possible using 1 mL of dissolution medium. However, the evaluation of both LMWS and HMWS levels over the dissolution test showed a difference between both volumes. Indeed, the HMWS levels were higher with 3DP_45 (5 mL) (Fig. 74e) after 6 weeks than observed with 3DP_44 (1 mL) (Fig. 77) (25.4 ± 3.6% *vs* 8.3 ± 1.1%). The dissolution test was performed in the same conditions (i.e. 37 °C, stirring at 600 rpm, PBS solution pH 7.0) except for the volume, which was increased from 1 mL to 5 mL. As previously shown, the lower volume (i.e. 1 mL) was assumed to be more destructive, with a higher pH drop observed after 6 weeks. The hypothesis is that harsh conditions may directly degrade the mAb structure within the polymeric matrix and create insoluble aggregates. These insoluble aggregates could have remained in the polymeric matrix and might have not been quantified.

II.6 Stability study of mAb-loaded 3DP devices

The development of mAb-loaded 3DP devices was described for the first time in this chapter. As the evaluation of the stability of the drug during storage is needed when a DDS is developed, it seemed mandatory to investigate our devices. The formulation made of the Tre-Leu association with a mAb:stabilizer ratio at 2.0:1 showed promising results. Following the previous results, the 3DP devices batch (3DP_46) was produced to perform this stability study. These devices were obtained using the same quantities and parameters as described previously (Table 17).

The phase separation of PEG at room temperature (20 °C) and higher temperatures without or with desiccant was previously demonstrated (Table 14, experimental part II section III.2.1). However, the stability of the mAb or the polymeric degradation over time have not yet been discussed.

This study focused only on the effect of storage temperatures on the stability of the mAb and the PLGA derivatives. Two temperatures were used, 5 ± 3 °C and 25 ± 2 °C, corresponding to cold storage (i.e. fridge) and room temperature, which may also be considered as stressed conditions for such polymeric implantable systems. The study lasted 6 months with intermediate points (T0, T1, T2, T3 and T6 months). 3DP devices (3DP_46) were produced using the mAb stabilized with the Tre-Leu association (Table 17) and were introduced in Fiolax® glass vials (Schott, DE) that were hermetically sealed with Lyotec® stoppers (West Pharmaceutical Service, USA) to carry out the stability tests. The glass vials were sealed under nitrogen atmosphere. Indeed, the relative humidity was reported as deleterious to polyesters due to their susceptibility to hydrolysis. This study was performed to evaluate the thermodynamic stability of the system (e.g. T_g,) as well as the influence of storage temperature on the mAb release profile and its stability. In parallel, the evolution of the Mw of PLGA was also evaluated by GPC at each time point.

II.6.1 Physical state of polymeric matrix

DSC analyses of the 3DP devices were performed at different time points (Table 21). As previously mentioned, PLGA was plasticized using PEG 2 kDa at 11% (w/w) and the T_g of the filament was 21.8 ± 0.4 °C. After printing, the T_g remained similar at 20.7 ± 0.3 °C.

No increase in the T_g was observed over 3 months for both storage temperatures (i.e. 5 °C and 25 °C). However, an increase in the T_g to 29.7 ± 0.3 °C was observed after 6 months at 25 °C (Table 21). The T_g of the devices remained constant over 6 months at 5 °C. Moreover, minor melting peaks were observed on samples stored at 25 °C for 2 months (T2), 3 months (T3) and

6 months (T6). The T_m were observed at 45.2 ± 1.4 °C (T2), 45.9 ± 0.8 °C (T3) and 46.7 ± 0.4 °C (T6) (Table 21). The melting peak could be attributed to the presence of PEG, which was able to diffuse out of the polymeric matrix at a temperature higher than T_g of the polymer (i.e. 25 °C). The melting enthalpy of these melting peaks were recorded and showed an increase over months from 1.7 ± 0.9 J/g (T2) to 7.4 ± 0.6 J/g (T6). The increase in the melting enthalpy demonstrated a potential phase separation, with the PLGA chain mobility at 25 °C. After 2 and 3 months, the melting enthalpy remained low and the plasticizing effect was effective. The increase in the T_g after 6 months at 25 °C was associated with a higher value of the melting enthalpy, which was consistent with a phase separation between PLGA and PEG. The melting enthalpy of neat PEG was recorded around 193.4 J/g (data not shown). Therefore, only a small amount of the PEG seemed to be separated from the PLGA blend over 6 months. Similar observations were observed during a polymer ageing study. It was reported that PEG derivatives were able to crystallize over time due to an elevation of storage temperature and humidity [246]. The crystallization of the PEG derivatives may increase the stiffness of the devices and modify their mechanical and release properties [170,247].

Table 21. 3DP devices (3DP_46) printed to perform the stability study using the time points (T0, T1, T2, T3, T6) with their characteristics, such as glass transition temperature (T_g), PEG melting temperature (T_m) and melting enthalpy (ΔHm), and PLGA molecular weight (Mw).

Storage temperature (°C)	Time point	T_g (°C)	T_m (°C)	ΔHm (J/g)	Mw (kDa)
	T0	20.7 ± 0.3	/	/	17.2 ± 0.4
5	T1	20.6 ± 1.0	/	/	17.1 ± 0.2
	T2	20.2 ± 1.0	/	/	17.0 ± 0.1
	T3	20.5 ± 0.2	/	/	17.1 ± 0.2
	T6	20.4 ± 1.0	/	/	14.7 ± 0.1
25	T1	20.6 ± 1.2	/	/	17.0 ± 0.1
	T2	20.1 ± 0.9	45.2 ± 1,4	1.7 ± 0.9	16.7 ± 0.4
	T3	21.3 ± 1.8	45.9 ± 0.8	2.6 ± 2.1	16.6 ± 0.1
	T6	29.7 ± 0.3	46.7 ± 0.4	7.4 ± 0.6	13.3 ± 0.6

The degradation of the PLGA was assessed using GPC. Its Mw at T0 was found to be 17.02 ± 0.38 kDa, which was consistent with that of raw PLGA (Mw: 17.05 ± 0.45 kDa). No degradation occurred over 3 months of storage, regardless of the temperature. However, the result obtained for T6 samples were stored in a fridge for 1.5 months before measurement and this storage may affect the Mw of the polymer. It was assumed that the stability of the polymer was maintained at both storage temperatures, but further investigations are needed.

II.6.2 Visual assessment of the devices over storage time

Visual assessment was carried out on the 3DP devices stored at 5 °C and 25 °C (Fig. 79). No difference was shown for the devices stored at 5 °C over 6 months (Fig. 79a, b, c). Sticky samples were observed when devices were stored at 25 °C. Devices adhered to the bottom of glass vial but no loss of material was observed during the withdrawal step. This observation was found for every device stored at 25 °C, from T_1 to T_6 (Fig. 79.d, e, f). Moreover, the samples stored at 25 °C showed a deformation of their shapes. Such bending is likely to be due to the position of the device inside the vial and was associated to the storage temperature, which was higher than its T_g. Indeed, the soft state of the material due to the increase in mobility of the chains of the polymer, as well as the effect of the gravity, led to the devices bending. The handling of the devices demonstrated an increase in their brittleness during the storage. It was assumed that this behaviour was due to the phase separation between PEG and PLGA. The cross-section of the devices after 6 months at 25 °C showed a highly porous network (Fig. 79g).

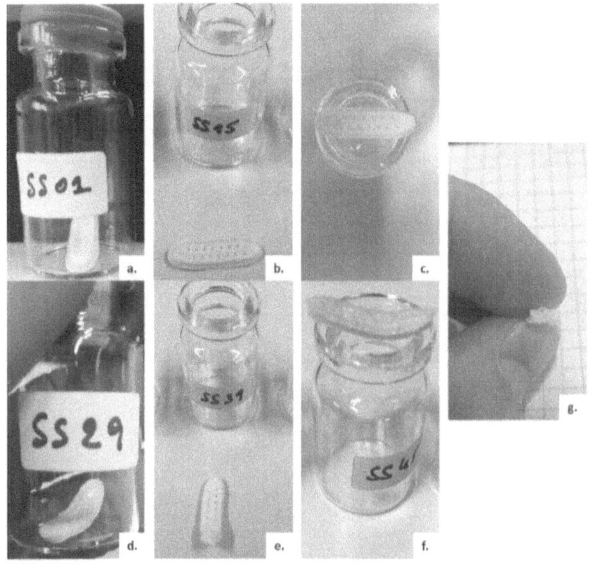

Fig. 79. Photographs of the 3DP specimens during storage: (**a.**) 1 month (T_1), (**b.**) 3 months (T_3) and (**c.**) 6 months (T_6) at 5 °C; (**d.**) T_1, (**e.**) T_3 and (**f.**) T_6 at 25 °C; and (**g.**) a cross-section of a device from T_6 at 25 °C.

II.6.3 mAb content and degradation

The quantification of the mAb from the devices was performed by BCA after extraction from the devices. The theoretical loading was 15% (w/w). As could be observed, the storage temperature did not influence the mAb loading as these loadings were $15.4 \pm 0.2\%$ and $15.4 \pm 0.3\%$ at 5 °C and 25 °C after 6 months, respectively (Table 22).

Table 22. Comparison of the mAb loading (%), the monomer content (%) and the HMWS and LMWS levels (%) according to storage time points, from T_0 (reference) to T_6 (6 months).

Storage temperature (°C)	Time point	mAb loading (%)	Monomer content (%)	HMWS level (%)	LMWS level (%)
	T0	15.4 ± 0.5	95.3 ± 0.2	4.7 ± 0.2	0.02 ± 0.02
5	T1	15.3 ± 0.3	95.7 ± 0.2	4.3 ± 0.2	0.05 ± 0.05
5	T2	16.1 ± 0.3	95.9 ± 0.3	4.0 ± 0.3	0.03 ± 0.06
5	T3	16.1 ± 0.2	95.4 ± 0.2	4.6 ± 0.2	0
5	T6	15.4 ± 0.2	95.7 ± 0.1	4.3 ± 0.1	0.08 ± 0.01
25	T1	15.3 ± 0.4	95.6 ± 0.3	4.4 ± 0.3	0
25	T2	15.5 ± 0.2	95.3 ± 0.3	4.7 ± 0.3	0.03 ± 0.05
25	T3	15.8 ± 0.3	95.7 ± 1.3	4.3 ± 1.3	0
25	T6	15.4 ± 0.3	94.8 ± 0.2	5.1 ± 0.2	0.08 ± 0.01

*LMWS: 0 correspond to a value below the limit of detection.

The stability of the mAb was assessed at each time point. The monomer content remained stable over 6 months at 5 °C. However, a slight decrease in the monomer percentage was observed after 6 months at 25 °C (Table 22). This decrease was associated to a slight increase in both HMWS (5.1 ± 0.2%) and, to a lesser extent, LMWS (0.08 ± 0.01%) levels of the samples (Table 22). This low increase may be correlated to the mobility of the polymer chains over 6 months at 25 °C. The phase separation between PEG and PLGA may lead to the migration of the mAb. The diffusion of the mAb could form clusters which increase its instability due to the decrease in the distance between mAb molecules.

II.6.4 Dissolution test and binding capacity evaluation

The release of the mAb was observed over 6 weeks using the 3DP devices at T_0 (reference), T_3 and T_6 (Fig. 80). These results were generated using the former dissolution test conditions using a volume of 1 mL of PBS (as described in 'Materials and methods' – section II.4.2)

At the lowest storage temperature, the burst effect observed from devices stored at 5 °C remained quite limited and remained steady over 6 months. Indeed, the burst effect observed at T_6 was 1.2 ± 0.1% and was similar to that obtained from the reference T_0 (1.4 ± 0.2%).

However, at 25 °C, the burst release from the devices after 3 and 6 months was notably increased in comparison with the devices stored at 5 °C. The burst effect observed at T_3 and T_6

were 17.1 ± 6.6% and 19.1 ± 2.8%, respectively (Fig. 80). The increase in the burst effect at 25 °C may be correlated with the phase separation and the migration of the PEG to the surface of the devices. The hydrophilic behaviour of PEG increased the diffusion of the water and thus, increased the release of the mAb.

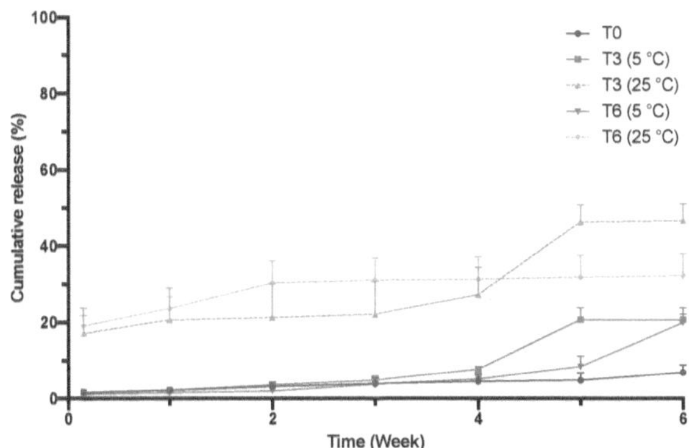

Fig. 80. Dissolution profiles of the mAb after time points T_0, T_3 and T_6 at both storage temperatures (**a**) 5 °C and (**b**) 25 °C (n=3, mean ± SD).

The cumulative release of the mAb from all samples, from T_0 to T_6 at 5 °C, showed the same trend with a slight difference between release patterns. However, differences in terms of release were observed after 4 weeks (Fig. 80a.). The erosion of the polymeric matrix was reported to start after 4 weeks, as previously discussed. Although no physical state changes were observed for these samples, the release was enhanced after 3 and 6 months to reach 38.5 ± 14.5% and 32.2 ± 5.7%, respectively.

The similarity factor f2 between the dissolution profiles was assessed. It was demonstrated these were similar for T_0, T_3 and T_6, with storage at 5 °C (f2 > 50). An f2 value higher than 50 for the release profiles before and after storage indicated that 3DP devices remained stable at 5 °C. At 25 °C, the dissolution profiles showed higher differences with the devices at T0, with an f2 value lower than 50. It was assumed that such difference was mainly due to the modification of the physical state and the higher porosity of the devices at the early stage of the release.

These release profiles were quite different from those previously observed with 3DP_44 (Fig. 72, section II.5). The burst release was lower with T_0 (1.4 ± 0.2%) than 3DP_44 (6.1 ± 0.5%). Furthermore, the cumulative releases after 6 weeks were 63.2 ± 4.7% and 6.9 ± 2.0% with 3DP_44 and T_0, respectively. These results were unexpected given the use of the same formulation, with the same processing methods and dissolution test parameters. One hypothesis could be related to the degradation of PLGA matrix over time with a volume of 1 mL of PBS. Further investigations (i.e. as previously performed with a volume of 5 mL (section II.5.2.1)) are therefore needed to evaluate the PLGA degradation kinetics.

Finally, the relative binding capacity of the mAb was assessed for the sample collected after 24h of dissolution and compared with the concentration obtained by UV detection (Fig. 81). The binding capacity of the mAb seemed to be fully preserved after 24h of release, regardless of the storage temperature. According to the results obtained by ELISA, the binding remained steady over 6 months. Further characterizations should be required to improve our knowledge of the stability and remaining activity of the mAb.

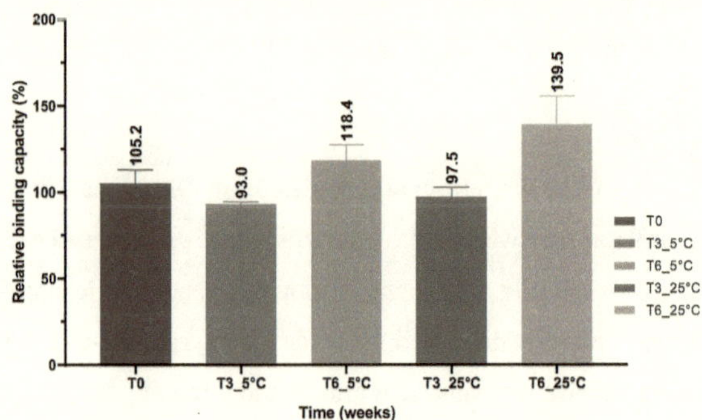

Fig. 81. Comparison of the relative binding capacity of mAb after 24h of release from 3DP devices, the reference time, and T_3 and T_6, stored at 5 °C and 25 °C.

III.   **Conclusion**

Our results showed that the association of HME and an FDM 3D printer was suitable to produce mAb-loaded DDS. Homogeneous solid dispersion of the mAb (with a loading of 15% (w/w)) in the PLGA matrix was reached in both printable filaments and 3DP DDS. Different stabilizers were investigated to stabilize the mAb against thermal degradation. Disaccharides (Tre and Suc) promoted mAb integrity during the SD, HME and 3DP steps using an mAb:stabilizer ratio of 2.0:1. The optimization of the formulation using a low amount of Leu (5% (w/w)) allowed stabilizing the mAb against potential thermal degradation. The association of mAb with Tre-Leu showed the lowest HMWS levels and no fragmentation was observed after 3DP. The dissolution profile showed an interesting sustained-release profile with a limited burst effect. However, the 3DP devices with similar compositions demonstrated variability in terms of release profiles. Finally, it was demonstrated that, despite the relatively high temperatures of extrusion (90 °C) and printing (105 °C), mAb binding capacity of up to 70% was maintained after 24h of dissolution. However, preliminary investigation of similar 3DP DDS showed a binding capacity around 90%. This observation was compared with the HMWS and LMWS levels during the mAb dissolution from the 3DP DDS. The monomer content demonstrated a value of 96.5 ± 0.3% after 24h. Thus, complementary analytical methods may be necessary to understand how thermal stresses impair the mAb binding capacity.

This study performed on the 3DP DDS showed that stability was ensured at 5 °C up to 6 months of storage. The release of the mAb and the mAb binding capacity remained stable at 5 °C, while degradation occurred at 25 °C. The polymeric matrix was reported to be thermodynamically stable at 5 °C and no degradation of the PLGA was observed, regardless the storage temperature (i.e. 5 °C and 25 °C). The release of the mAb showed a higher burst release when devices stored at 25 °C were used. The phase separation between the PEG and the PLGA could explained that a faster release was observed. Finally, the binding capacity of the mAb was preserved over the 6 months of stability test.

Further *in vivo* investigations may be useful to complete and correlate the *in vitro* data generated in this work.

Part IV – Evaluation and development of 3DP DDS containing a monoclonal antibody fragment

I. Introduction

The development of mAb-loaded 3DP devices was successfully achieved. However, mAb are usually characterized by a plasma half-life of 11-30 days [248]. Our model was developed to ensure a sustained release of the biotherapeutic compounds. However, mAb elimination from the blood circulation is a slow phase, which leads to a long residence time and a risk of accumulation. Consequently, a monoclonal antibody fragment (Fab) was identified to be more adapted to perform a proof of concept. Indeed, it was previously reported that the plasma half-life of a 50 kDa Fab fragment was around 28 min [249]. The Fab model was therefore the most suitable to produce a sustained-release DDS in order to extend its half-life [250].

This section describes the preliminary results obtained on a Fab model provided by UCB Pharma. As mentioned previously, formulations containing disaccharides such as Tre or Suc showed interesting results for stabilizing our mAb model. Both stabilizers, with and without the addition of Leu, were used to develop and evaluate for 3DP DDS when a Fab was loaded.

II. Results and discussion

II.1 Development of Fab-loaded 3DP DDS

The Fab formulation was performed using BE. No instabilities were found between the initial Fab reference solution and the BE step, following the technique described in 'Materials and methods' – section II.1.1c. The Fab reference solution (provided by UCB Pharma) was characterized with a monomer content and a HMWS level of 99.6 ± 0.2% and 0.4 ± 0.2%, respectively. The Fab was more stable than the mAb previously used. Indeed, the mAb reference solution showed a monomer content of 97.4 ± 0.4% and HMWS level of 2.6 ± 0.4% (Table 18). The formulation of the Fab contained Tre or Suc, with or without Leu, to compare four different formulations and determine which one could stabilize it the most against thermal stresses. All the formulations were produced using a Fab:stabilizer ratio of 2.0:1 (Table 23).

The Fab was spray-dried and the yield of SD was higher than expected. As discussed previously, a range between 50 and 70% (w/w) was expected when biotherapeutics are dried using SD [161]. The spray-dried powders were characterized by a yield between 85.5% (SDFF_3) and 91.1% (SDFF_2) (Table 23). Consequently, the selected parameters based on our in-house protocol (as described in 'Materials and methods' – section II.1.2b) seemed adapted to the Fab as well.

The filaments were produced using the same parameters previously used to produce mAb-filament using HME (Process 11, ThermoFisher Scientific, USA) (as described in 'Materials and methods' – section II.2.2). These filaments were loaded with a theoretical loading of 15% (w/w) which was previously selected when mAb-loaded filaments were prepared (as decribed in part III section II.3). According to the use of optimized parameters on HME, all the filaments were prepared with a diameter between 1.70 and 1.75 mm, as required for further printing [71].

Finally, the printable filaments were used to feed the Hyrel 30M system 3D printer (Hyrel®, USA) and produce devices. The devices were designed using ThinkerCad (Autodesk®, USA) and printed using a temperature of 105 °C, an infill density of 100% and a layer thickness of 0.3 mm (as described in 'Materials and methods' – section II.3.3).

Table 23. Theoretical composition of evaluated Fab formulations for spray-dried batches (% w/V), solid composition of spray-dried powders (% w/w) and the yield of the SD process (%), printable filaments produced using HME batches (% w/w) with the yield of the process (%) and associated 3DP batches printed with an infill density of 100% (v/v) and 0.3 mm of layer thickness (n=3).

SD batch number	Stab.	Fab:stab. ratio	His	Stab.	Leu	Fab	His	Stab.	Leu	Fab	SD yield (%)	HME batch number	RG502 (% w/w)	PEG (% w/w)	Excipient (% w/w)	Fab (% w/w)	HME yield (%)	3DP batch number
			Liquid composition (% w/V) - after BE				Solid composition (% w/w) - after spray drying											
SDFF_1	Suc		0.2	3.8	-	8.0	1.9	31.4	-	66.7	87.9	HME_F_1	69.4	7.6	7.6	15.3	58.3	3DP_F_1
SDFF_2	Suc-Leu	2.0:1	0.2	3.2	0.6	8.0	1.9	26.4	5.0	66.7	91.1	HME_F_2	69.4	7.6	7.6	15.3	57.8	3DP_F_2
SDFF_3	Tre		0.2	3.8	-	8.0	1.9	31.4	-	66.7	85.5	HME_F_3	69.4	7.6	7.6	15.3	56,0	3DP_F_3
SDFF_4	Tre-Leu		0.2	3.2	0.6	8.0	1.9	26.4	5.0	66.7	89.5	HME_F_4	69.4	7.6	7.6	15.3	55.9	3DP_F_4

*(Stab.: stabilizer)

The stability of the Fab was evaluated using the formation of HMWS. After SD, there was no significant formation of HMWS, regardless of the formulation (p-value > 0.05) (Fig. 82). Afterwards, the Fab was extracted from polymeric matrix of both printable filaments and 3DP devices after HME and FDM, respectively. The Fab extracted was compared with the related spray-dried powder in terms of HMWS level (Fig. 82). It was demonstrated that the level of HMWS of the formulated Fab slightly increased after HME and 3DP. For instance, the HMWS level of formulation containing Tre-Leu evolved from 0.6 ± 0.3% after SD to 1.0 ± 0.1% after 3DP (Fig. 82). It was observed that the HMWS level increased from 0.5 ± 0.5% (SD) to 0.7 ± 0.1% (3DP) when Suc-Leu were used as stabilizers. Furthermore, no LMWS were observed, which indicated that no fragmentation occurred despite the high process temperatures. According to these results, none of the formulations were significantly different from the Fab-spray-dried powder (p-value > 0.05).

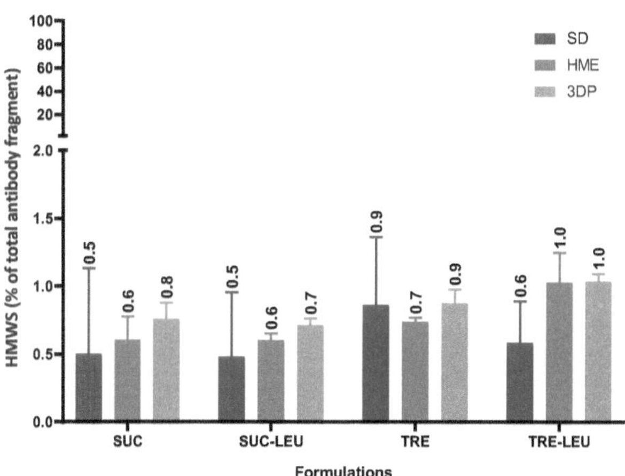

Fig. 82. Comparison of the HMWS levels for the Fab formulation (Fab:stabilizer ratio 2.0:1) containing Suc, Suc-Leu, Tre and Tre-Leu after SD, HME and 3DP (n = 3, mean ± SD). The Fab reference was characterized with a monomer content and a HMWS level of 99.6 ± 0.2% and 0.4 ± 0.2%, respectively.

*Formulations are summarized as SUC: SD_F_1 (SD), HME_F_1 (HME), 3DP_F_1 (3DP); SUC-LEU: SD_F_2 (SD), HME_F_2 (HME), 3DP_F_2 (3DP); TRE: SD_F_3 (SD), HME_F_3 (HME), 3DP_F_3 (3DP); TRE-LEU: SD_F_4 (SD), HME_F_4 (HME), 3DP_F_4 (3DP) Table 23.

II.2 Dissolution test

A dissolution study was performed on all printed devices to investigate both the dissolution profiles and the stability of the Fab over the release time (Fig. 83). The dissolution tests were performed using the optimized conditions (i.e. volume of 5 mL) used to carry out the dissolution on 3DP_45 (as described in experimental part III - section II.5.2). The burst effects from all devices were limited, regardless of the formulation. For instance, the highest burst release value only reached 2.4 ± 0.2% (3DP_F_4) after 24h. These burst releases were quite similar to the value obtained with the mAb, which was 2.3 ± 0.3% (Fig. 76a).

As previously observed, triphasic profiles were obtained from all devices. This observation was mainly dependent on the monolithic state of the device and the difficulty of the dissolution medium to diffuse into it. A phase of slow release was observed between weeks 1 and 4, with values of 5.3 ± 0.7% (3DP_F_1), 5.4 ± 0.7% (3DP_F_2), 6.4 ± 1.3% (3DP_F_3) and 6.3 ± 0.5% (3DP_F_4). As previously explained, the degradation of the polymer increased after 3 weeks due to erosion (as decribed in experimental part III - section II.5.2.1). Consequently, a faster release was observed between weeks 4 and 7. These results support the previous results obtained with mAb-loaded 3DP DDS (Fig. 76a). Finally, a maximal cumulative release of 79.3 ± 14.7% was observed from device 3DP_F_4 after 8 weeks (Fig. 83). The maximal cumulative release of each Fab-loaded 3DP device was higher than those observed with the mAb-loaded devices after 8 weeks. This result could be due to the smaller Mw of the Fab model (~ 50 kDa *vs* 150 kDa), which allowed easier diffusion from the polymeric matrix to the dissolution medium through the porous network.

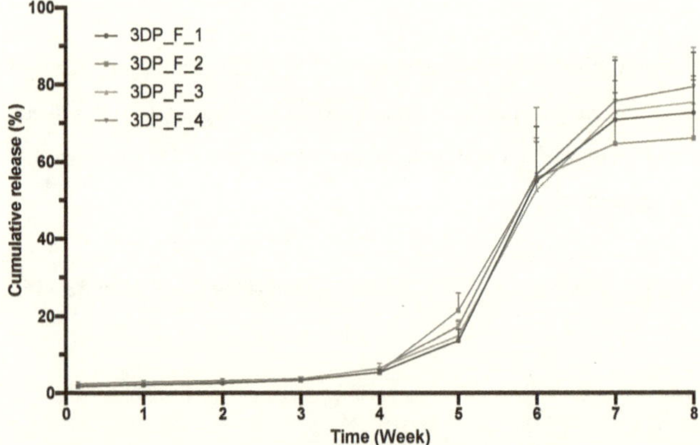

Fig. 83. In vitro dissolution profiles of 3DP DDS containing Fab stabilized with Suc (3DP_F_1), Suc-Leu (3DP_F_2), Tre (3DP_F_3) and Tre-Leu formulations (3DP_F_4).

II.2.1 Fab stability over release

During the dissolution test, both monomer content and HMWS levels were investigated over 8 weeks. A slight decrease in monomer content was observed after 8 weeks. Indeed, the monomer content decreased from $99.3 \pm 0.1\%$ to $97.6 \pm 1.0\%$ with 3DP_F_4 (Fig. 84a). After 2 weeks of dissolution, a deformation of the monomer peak on the SEC result was observed (data not shown). A shoulder appeared on the monomer peak and increased over weeks, but no fragmentation was observed after 8 weeks, regardless of the formulation (data not shown). Such shoulder on a SEC chromatogram may be explained by the acidic microclimate in the PLGA matrix, which impaired the Fab integrity.

An increase in the HMWS level was demonstrated (Fig. 84b). The aggregation of the Fab during its dissolution seemed limited in comparison to the previous results observed for the mAb. For instance, the percentage of HMWS from 3DP_F_4, after 8 weeks of dissolution, was $1.9 \pm 0.1\%$. No fragmentation of the Fab was observed (data not shown). The Fab and the mAb were two different molecules in terms of M_w or stability, which was intrinsically related to the molecule. The Fab seemed to be more stable when similar conditions were applied. Indeed, the aggregation of the Fab over the weeks was quite low after HME and 3DP as well as during the dissolution test, regardless of the formulation selected.

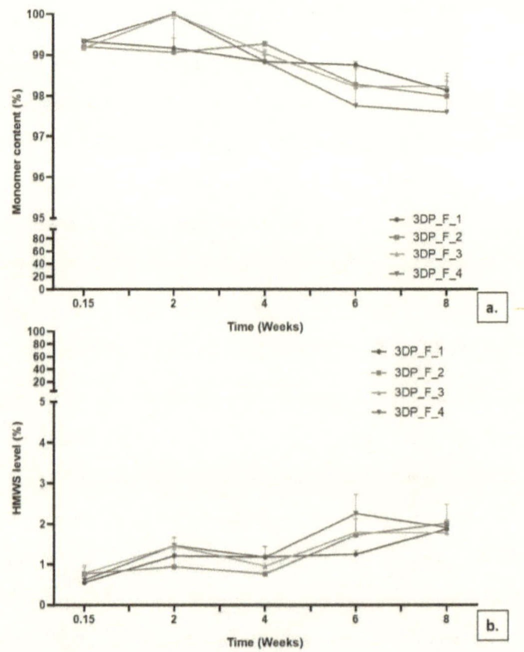

Fig. 84. Comparison of the monomer content (**a**) and HMWS levels (**b**) of Fab released from 3DP_F_1 (Suc), 3DP_F_2 (Suc-Leu), 3DP_F_3 (Tre) and 3DP_F_4 (Tre-Leu) over the dissolution time up to 8 weeks.

II.2.2 Binding capacity of the Fab

The binding capacity of the Fab was assessed to confirm that it was able to successively bind to its target. ELISA data demonstrated that the binding capacity of the Fab was preserved after 24h of release, regardless of the formulation. For instance, the binding capacity of 3DP_F_4 was 99.5 ± 6.4% (Fig. 85). These results suggested that all formulations were adapted to successively dry the Fab, produce printable filaments and print the 3DP devices with a limited degradation of the fragment.

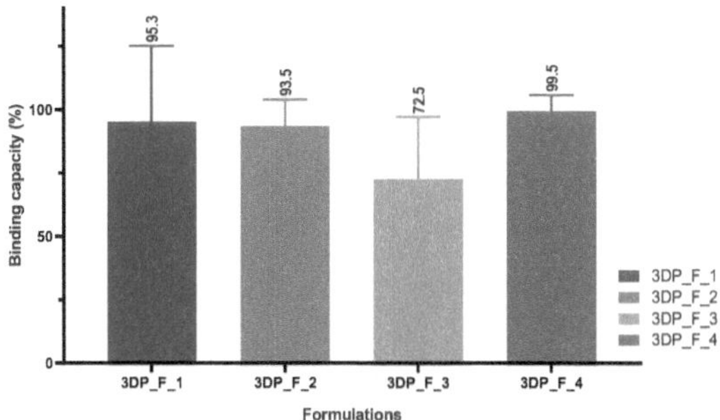

Fig. 85. Binding capacity of the Fab released from 3DP_F_1, 3DP_F_2, 3DP_F_3 and 3DP_F_4 after 24h of dissolution.

III.   Conclusion

To conclude this part, the 3DP DDS developed for both pIgG and then mAb was successfully applied to a third biological entity. The Fab was successively dried, extruded and printed using four different formulations containing Suc or Tre, with or without Leu. The 3DP devices allowed a sustained release of the Fab over 8 weeks. Besides, the HMWS level remained low with a maximum value of 1.9 ± 0.1% (3DP_F_4). These results gave consistency to the feasibility of using biotherapeutics in drastic thermal processes such as HME and FDM. This preliminary study conducted on the Fab model showed promising results that seemed better than those observed with mAb in terms of stability, release and binding capacity. Finally, the study focused on aggregation and/or fragmentation using HMWS and LMWS to determine the integrity of Fab. Further investigations, as previously mentioned, are needed to improve the knowledge on structural changes on Fab structure. Finally, an *in vivo* study may confirm all these statements on the stability, release and binding capacity over time with the determination of pharmacokinetic parameters such as the maximum concentration peak, maximum time-to-peak concentration, half-life, or elimination constant.

General conclusion and perspectives

This project aimed to produce antibody-loaded 3DP IDDS which should be able to promote a sustained release of the loaded biotherapeutic. The main novelty of this project was the implementation of the FDM technology to develop such devices. To our knowledge, this work was the first which reported the development of this kind of platform. Three different biological entities (i.e. pIgG, mAb and Fab) were investigated during this project to evaluate the robustness of the method. Furthermore, the use of HME and FDM allowed producing high drug loading IDDS ($\geq$ 15% (w/w)).

The first part of the project was mainly oriented to the investigation of the mechanical properties of the printed devices and to the evaluation of the influence of the printing parameters on both printing process and quality of the devices. A DoE approach was performed to evaluated different types of plasticizers (i.e. TA, ATEC, PEG400 and TEC) on the processability of PLA matrix. It was demonstrated that the stiffness of the PLA was lowered when using ATEC and the adhesion between layers was promoted when TA was added. Moreover, the ductility of the material was improved when a higher layer thickness was fixed. During this study, the deposition temperature of PLA was successfully decreased from 230 °C to 190, 173 and 155 °C. The decrease in the deposition temperature was performed with the addition of 10% (w/w) of plasticizer. These results showed the opportunity to lower the deposition temperature and thus, the possibility of loading a thermosensitive drug compound inside the printable filament.

The development of a printable filament containing a pIgG model was investigated. This pIgG was available in large amounts and affordable, in comparison with a mAb for instance. It was quickly decided to focus our research on the use of biodegradable and biocompatible polymers such as PLGA derivatives. The selection of the raw PLGA derivatives was performed on three types of PLGA, which were characterized by different Mw such as PDLG 5004 (Mw: 44 kDa) and RG502 (Mw: 7-17 kDa). One type was a PEG-PLGA block copolymer (2 kDa-20 kDa). The latter was selected to be compared with plasticized PLGA using free PEG 2kDa to enhance the processability and to improve the physical behaviour of the PLGA. Indeed, the extrusion temperature was a key parameter in incorporating an antibody into a hot melted polymeric matrix. Printable filaments were successfully extruded using three types of PLGA matrix. The filaments were used to feed the 3D printer and to produce 3DP devices. However, it was demonstrated that high temperatures were mainly responsible for pIgG degradation. PLGA RG502 was selected for further experiments because it may be extruded at 90 °C and printed at 113 °C when a plasticizer (PEG 2kDa) is added. The preliminary dissolution tests showed a limited burst release after 24h of dissolution and a sustained release over time. This part of the study showed the opportunity to develop pIgG-loaded 3DP devices using FDM technology.

The optimization of the printable filament was necessary to enhance its homogeneity as well as its brittleness. It was demonstrated that the addition of 11% (w/w) of PEG 2kDa to the PLGA matrix led to suitable physical properties and minimized the waste of material. The blending conditions were improved to promote a homogeneous dispersion of the pIgG into the PLGA matrix through the whole length of the filament. Then, the evaluation of the influence of some printing parameters on the final physicochemical properties of the 3DP devices, such as the deposition temperature, the layer thickness and the infill density, were carried out. The influence of the deposition temperature on the release profile of the loaded pIgG was demonstrated. Indeed, the increase in the deposition temperature from 113 °C to 115 °C showed a slower release of the pIgG over time. This observation may be due to the less porous structure of the matrix when the deposition temperature was increased. However, the pIgG model starting material was characterized with initial high levels of both HMWS and LMWS. Therefore, the potential degradation that could be generated during the processing methods may be hidden.

The selected processing methods were applied to a mAb model provided by UCB Pharma. To develop these 3DP IDDS, the formulation of the mAb was developed using several stabilizers at three different mAb:stabilizer ratios. The selection of the stabilizers and the ratio was performed according the evaluation of both HMWS and LMWS levels after each step of production. The mAb was formulated and dried using SD. It has been widely accepted that proteins in a solid state are more stable. It was demonstrated that a mAb:stabilizer ratio of 2.0:1 using Tre and Suc was effective in stabilizing the mAb during melt encapsulation. Both compounds (Suc and Tre) are characterized by similar structure, which belongs to the disaccharide class. It has already been noted that such derivatives are able to create hydrogen bonds with the protein. They also form a glassy matrix to avoid protein-protein interactions, which are known to avoid aggregation issues. The ability of both disaccharides to minimize the formation of aggregates and to avoid the fragmentation of the mAb was demonstrated over this study after HME and 3DP. A higher stability was reached using a combination of these disaccharides with 5% (w/w) of Leu. The formulation containing the Tre-Leu association was able to minimize the aggregation of the mAb. The improvement of the 3DP step using a 3D printer with a modular print head allowed decreasing the deposition temperature to 105 °C. The sustained release of the mAb was demonstrated as well as the evolution of the erosion of the system according to the progressive decrease in the Mw of the PLGA over the dissolution study. The integrity of the mAb was assessed over weeks during the dissolution test and a decrease in the monomer content was shown. However, the decrease in the pH in the dissolution medium and the erosion of the PLGA led to an increase in both HMWS and LMWS levels. Nonetheless, the binding capacity of the mAb was preserved after the successive processing methods.

A stability study was performed on the mAb-loaded 3D IDDS to assess PLGA matrix and mAb degradation. The 3DP devices were stable at a storage temperature of 5 °C. The PLGA matrix remained stable at 5 °C while at 25 °C a phase separation between PEG and PLGA was reported. The 3DP devices stored at 25 °C were shown to be bent due to the low T_g of the polymeric matrix. The properties of the matrix were preserved at 5 °C and the dissolution profiles remained similar. The 3DP devices stored at 25 °C demonstrated an increase in the burst release. The binding affinity of the mAb was shown to be preserved during storage at both temperatures after 24h of dissolution.

Finally, the optimized processing methods were applied with success to a Fab fragment. This study showed that the selected stabilizers, such as Tre and Suc, with or without Leu, were adapted to stabilize our Fab model. The HMWS levels were lower than those observed from the devices containing the mAb. It seemed that the Fab was less affected by the production method . The feasibility and the applicability of FDM technology to print IDDS loaded with a biotherapeutic was demonstrated. The sustained release of the loaded antibody was observed for three different biologic entities. The next step of this work should be a further *in vivo* study on rodents to assess the release of the Fab from the IDDS and its biodistribution. A comparison between an immediate-release formulation of Fab using the intravenous or subcutaneous routes and the Fab-loaded 3DP IDDS should be performed. This approach may validate the concept and confirm the sustained release of the Fab over time, as shown during the *in vitro* dissolution tests.

To conclude, the 3DP of IDDS containing biotherapeutics was shown to be effective. However, according to the generated results, it should be interesting to investigate more deeply the antibody structure. Indeed, the main concern on antibody therapy remains its structural stability and degradation products must be fully investigated to avoid any adverse effects. Analytical method such as circular dichroism and fluorescence spectroscopy as well as nuclear magnetic resonance may be useful to characterize the secondary and tertiary structures of the antibody after these drastic processes. The acidification of the medium during the dissolution test led to the degradation of the mAb. These degradations may occur on both Fab and Fc regions of the mAb which leads to a decreased biological activity. Degradation of the antibody leads to immunogenicity and reduce its efficacy as well as the safety that cause anti-drug antibody responses and hypersensitivity reactions. The knowledge on how mAb (or Fab) degrades could therefore help to optimize the formulation and promote a further stability.

REFERENCES

[1]   J. Goole, K. Amighi, 3D printing in pharmaceutics: A new tool for designing customized drug delivery systems, Int. J. Pharm. 499 (2016) 376–394. https://doi.org/10.1016/j.ijpharm.2015.12.071.

[2]   O. Abdulhameed, A. Al-Ahmari, W. Ameen, S.H. Mian, Additive manufacturing: Challenges, trends, and applications, Adv. Mech. Eng. 11 (2019) 168781401882288. https://doi.org/10.1177/1687814018822880.

[3]   J.L. Walker, M. Santoro, Processing and production of bioresorbable polymer scaffolds for tissue engineering, in: Bioresorbable Polym. Biomed. Appl. From Fundam. to Transl. Med., 2016: pp. 181–203. https://doi.org/10.1016/B978-0-08-100262-9.00009-4.

[4]   D.R. Eyers, A.T. Potter, Industrial Additive Manufacturing: A manufacturing systems perspective, Comput. Ind. 92–93 (2017) 208–218. https://doi.org/10.1016/j.compind.2017.08.002.

[5]   S.M.F. Kabir, K. Mathur, A.F.M. Seyam, A critical review on 3D printed continuous fiber-reinforced composites: History, mechanism, materials and properties, Compos. Struct. 232 (2020). https://doi.org/10.1016/j.compstruct.2019.111476.

[6]   B.C. Gross, J.L. Erkal, S.Y. Lockwood, C. Chen, D.M. Spence, Evaluation of 3D printing and its potential impact on biotechnology and the chemical sciences, Anal. Chem. 86 (2014) 3240–3253. https://doi.org/10.1021/ac403397r.

[7]   S. Lamichhane, S. Bashyal, T. Keum, G. Noh, J.E. Seo, R. Bastola, J. Choi, D.H. Sohn, S. Lee, Complex formulations, simple techniques: Can 3D printing technology be the Midas touch in pharmaceutical industry?, Asian J. Pharm. Sci. 14 (2019) 465–479. https://doi.org/10.1016/j.ajps.2018.11.008.

[8]   L. Zema, A. Melocchi, A. Maroni, A. Gazzaniga, Three-Dimensional Printing of Medicinal Products and the Challenge of Personalized Therapy, J. Pharm. Sci. 106 (2017) 1697–1705. https://doi.org/10.1016/j.xphs.2017.03.021.

[9]   A. Mohammed, A. Elshaer, P. Sareh, M. Elsayed, H. Hassanin, Additive Manufacturing Technologies for Drug Delivery Applications, Int. J. Pharm. 580 (2020). https://doi.org/10.1016/j.ijpharm.2020.119245.

[10]   G. Tiwari, R. Tiwari, S. Bannerjee, L. Bhati, S. Pandey, P. Pandey, B. Sriwastawa, Drug delivery systems: An updated review, Int. J. Pharm. Investig. 2 (2012) 2. https://doi.org/10.4103/2230-973x.96920.

[11]   R.A. Jain, The manufacturing techniques of various drug loaded biodegradable poly(lactide-co-glycolide) (PLGA) devices, Biomaterials. 21 (2000) 2475–2490. https://doi.org/10.1016/S0142-9612(00)00115-0.

[12]   W. Jamróz, J. Szafraniec, M. Kurek, R. Jachowicz, 3D Printing in Pharmaceutical and Medical Applications – Recent Achievements and Challenges, Springer New York LLC, 2018. https://doi.org/10.1007/s11095-018-2454-x.

[13]   S.J. Trenfield, A. Awad, A. Goyanes, S. Gaisford, A.W. Basit, 3D Printing Pharmaceuticals: Drug Development to Frontline Care, Trends Pharmacol. Sci. 39 (2018) 440–451. https://doi.org/10.1016/j.tips.2018.02.006.

[14]   A. Melocchi, M. Uboldi, A. Maroni, A. Foppoli, L. Palugan, L. Zema, A. Gazzaniga, 3D printing by fused

deposition modeling of single- and multi-compartment hollow systems for oral delivery – A review, Int. J. Pharm. 579 (2020) 119155. https://doi.org/10.1016/j.ijpharm.2020.119155.

[15] B.J. Park, H.J. Choi, S.J. Moon, S.J. Kim, R. Bajracharya, J.Y. Min, H.K. Han, Pharmaceutical applications of 3D printing technology: current understanding and future perspectives, J. Pharm. Investig. 49 (2019) 575–585. https://doi.org/10.1007/s40005-018-00414-y.

[16] L.K. Prasad, H. Smyth, 3D Printing technologies for drug delivery: a review, Drug Dev. Ind. Pharm. 9045 (2015) 1–13. https://doi.org/10.3109/03639045.2015.1120743.

[17] N. Sandler, M. Preis, Printed Drug-Delivery Systems for Improved Patient Treatment, Trends Pharmacol. Sci. 37 (2016) 1070–1080. https://doi.org/10.1016/j.tips.2016.10.002.

[18] A. Melocchi, F. Parietti, S. Maccagnan, M.A. Ortenzi, S. Antenucci, F. Briatico-Vangosa, A. Maroni, A. Gazzaniga, L. Zema, Industrial Development of a 3D-Printed Nutraceutical Delivery Platform in the Form of a Multicompartment HPC Capsule, AAPS PharmSciTech. 19 (2018) 3343–3354. https://doi.org/10.1208/s12249-018-1029-9.

[19] T. Feuerbach, S. Callau-Mendoza, M. Thommes, Development of filaments for fused deposition modeling 3D printing with medical grade poly(lactic-co-glycolic acid) copolymers, Pharm. Dev. Technol. 24 (2019) 487–493. https://doi.org/10.1080/10837450.2018.1514522.

[20] J. Norman, R.D. Madurawe, C.M.V. Moore, M.A. Khan, A. Khairuzzaman, A new chapter in pharmaceutical manufacturing: 3D-printed drug products, Adv. Drug Deliv. Rev. 108 (2017) 39–50. https://doi.org/10.1016/j.addr.2016.03.001.

[21] M. Trivedi, J. Jee, S. Silva, C. Blomgren, V.M. Pontinha, D.L. Dixon, B. Van Tassel, M.J. Bortner, C. Williams, E. Gilmer, A.P. Haring, J. Halper, B.N. Johnson, Z. Kong, M.S. Halquist, P.F. Rocheleau, T.E. Long, T. Roper, D.S. Wijesinghe, Additive manufacturing of pharmaceuticals for precision medicine applications: A review of the promises and perils in implementation, Addit. Manuf. 23 (2018) 319–328. https://doi.org/10.1016/j.addma.2018.07.004.

[22] J. Zhang, A.Q. Vo, X. Feng, S. Bandari, M.A. Repka, Pharmaceutical Additive Manufacturing: a Novel Tool for Complex and Personalized Drug Delivery Systems, AAPS PharmSciTech. 19 (2018) 3388–3402. https://doi.org/10.1208/s12249-018-1097-x.

[23] K. Shi, D.K. Tan, A. Nokhodchi, M. Maniruzzaman, Drop-On-Powder 3D printing of Tablets with an Anti-Cancer Drug, 5-Fluorouracil, Pharmaceutics. 11 (2019) 150. https://doi.org/10.3390/pharmaceutics11040150.

[24] T.D. Ngo, A. Kashani, G. Imbalzano, K.T.Q. Nguyen, D. Hui, Additive manufacturing (3D printing): A review of materials, methods, applications and challenges, Compos. Part B Eng. 143 (2018) 172–196. https://doi.org/10.1016/j.compositesb.2018.02.012.

[25] Aprecia Pharmaceuticals, ZipDose ® Technology, (2014) 1–2. https://www.aprecia.com/technology/zipdose (accessed March 21, 2017).

[26]   F. Fina, A. Goyanes, S. Gaisford, A.W. Basit, Selective laser sintering (SLS) 3D printing of medicines, Int. J. Pharm. 529 (2017) 285–293. https://doi.org/10.1016/j.ijpharm.2017.06.082.

[27]   R. Kolakovic, T. Viitala, P. Ihalainen, N. Genina, J. Peltonen, N. Sandler, Printing technologies in fabrication of drug delivery systems, Expert Opin. Drug Deliv. 10 (2013) 1711–1723. https://doi.org/10.1517/17425247.2013.859134.

[28]   M. Kyobula, A. Adedeji, M.R. Alexander, E. Saleh, R. Wildman, I. Ashcroft, P.R. Gellert, C.J. Roberts, 3D inkjet printing of tablets exploiting bespoke complex geometries for controlled and tuneable drug release, (2017). https://doi.org/10.1016/j.jconrel.2017.06.025.

[29]   X. Xu, P. Robles-Martinez, C.M. Madla, F. Joubert, A. Goyanes, A.W. Basit, S. Gaisford, Stereolithography (SLA) 3D printing of an antihypertensive polyprintlet: Case study of an unexpected photopolymer-drug reaction, Addit. Manuf. 33 (2020). https://doi.org/10.1016/j.addma.2020.101071.

[30]   M.A. Alhnan, T.C. Okwuosa, M. Sadia, K.W. Wan, W. Ahmed, B. Arafat, Emergence of 3D Printed Dosage Forms: Opportunities and Challenges, Pharm. Res. 33 (2016) 1817–1832. https://doi.org/10.1007/s11095-016-1933-1.

[31]   M.A. Azad, D. Olawuni, G. Kimbell, A.Z.M. Badruddoza, M.S. Hossain, T. Sultana, Polymers for extrusion-based 3D printing of pharmaceuticals: A holistic materials–process perspective, Pharmaceutics. 12 (2020) 124. https://doi.org/10.3390/pharmaceutics12020124.

[32]   S.A. Khaled, J.C. Burley, M.R. Alexander, J. Yang, C.J. Roberts, 3D printing of tablets containing multiple drugs with defined release profiles, Int. J. Pharm. 494 (2015) 643–650. https://doi.org/10.1016/j.ijpharm.2015.07.067.

[33]   S.A. Khaled, J.C. Burley, M.R. Alexander, J. Yang, C.J. Roberts, 3D printing of five-in-one dose combination polypill with defined immediate and sustained release profiles, J. Control. Release. 217 (2015) 308–314. https://doi.org/10.1016/j.jconrel.2015.09.028.

[34]   S.A. Khaled, J.C. Burley, M.R. Alexander, C.J. Roberts, Desktop 3D printing of controlled release pharmaceutical bilayer tablets, Int. J. Pharm. 461 (2014) 105–111. https://doi.org/10.1016/j.ijpharm.2013.11.021.

[35]   O.A. Mohamed, S.H. Masood, J.L. Bhowmik, Optimization of fused deposition modeling process parameters for dimensional accuracy using I-optimality criterion, Measurement. 81 (2016) 174–196. https://doi.org/10.1016/j.measurement.2015.12.011.

[36]   A.A. Konta, M. García-Piña, D.R. Serrano, Personalised 3D printed medicines: Which techniques and polymers are more successful?, Bioengineering. 4 (2017). https://doi.org/10.3390/bioengineering4040079.

[37]   A. Goyanes, A.B.M. Buanz, G.B. Hatton, S. Gaisford, A.W. Basit, 3D printing of modified-release aminosalicylate (4-ASA and 5-ASA) tablets, Eur. J. Pharm. Biopharm. 89 (2015) 157–162. https://doi.org/10.1016/j.ejpb.2014.12.003.

[38]   C.I. Gioumouxouzis, C. Karavasili, D.G. Fatouros, Recent advances in pharmaceutical dosage forms and devices using additive manufacturing technologies, Drug Discov. Today. 24 (2019) 636–643. https://doi.org/10.1016/j.drudis.2018.11.019.

[39]   A. Goyanes, A.B.M. Buanz, A.W. Basit, S. Gaisford, Fused-filament 3D printing (3DP) for fabrication of tablets, Int. J. Pharm. 476 (2014) 88–92. https://doi.org/10.1016/j.ijpharm.2014.09.044.

[40]   A. Goyanes, H. Chang, D. Sedough, G.B. Hatton, J. Wang, A. Buanz, S. Gaisford, A.W. Basit, Fabrication of controlled-release budesonide tablets via desktop (FDM) 3D printing, Int. J. Pharm. 496 (2015) 414–420. https://doi.org/10.1016/j.ijpharm.2015.10.039.

[41]   J. Skowyra, K. Pietrzak, M.A. Alhnan, Fabrication of extended-release patient-tailored prednisolone tablets via fused deposition modelling (FDM) 3D printing, Eur. J. Pharm. Sci. 68 (2015) 11–17. https://doi.org/10.1016/j.ejps.2014.11.009.

[42]   K. Pietrzak, A. Isreb, M.A. Alhnan, A flexible-dose dispenser for immediate and extended release 3D printed tablets, Eur. J. Pharm. Biopharm. 96 (2015) 380–387. https://doi.org/10.1016/j.ejpb.2015.07.027.

[43]   A. Goyanes, P. Robles Martinez, A. Buanz, A.W. Basit, S. Gaisford, Effect of geometry on drug release from 3D printed tablets, Int. J. Pharm. 494 (2015) 657–663. https://doi.org/10.1016/j.ijpharm.2015.04.069.

[44]   B. Arafat, N. Qinna, M. Cieszynska, R.T. Forbes, M.A. Alhnan, Tailored on demand anti-coagulant dosing: An in vitro and in vivo evaluation of 3D printed purpose-designed oral dosage forms, Eur. J. Pharm. Biopharm. 128 (2018) 282–289. https://doi.org/10.1016/j.ejpb.2018.04.010.

[45]   J. Fu, X. Yu, Y. Jin, 3D printing of vaginal rings with personalized shapes for controlled release of progesterone, Int. J. Pharm. 539 (2018) 75–82. https://doi.org/10.1016/j.ijpharm.2018.01.036.

[46]   J. Holländer, N. Genina, H. Jukarainen, M. Khajeheian, A. Rosling, E. M??kil??, N. Sandler, Three-Dimensional Printed PCL-Based Implantable Prototypes of Medical Devices for Controlled Drug Delivery, J. Pharm. Sci. 105 (2016) 2665–2676. https://doi.org/10.1016/j.xphs.2015.12.012.

[47]   N. Genina, J. Holländer, H. Jukarainen, E. Mäkilä, J. Salonen, N. Sandler, Ethylene vinyl acetate (EVA) as a new drug carrier for 3D printed medical drug delivery devices, Eur. J. Pharm. Sci. 90 (2016) 53–63. https://doi.org/10.1016/j.ejps.2015.11.005.

[48]   M.A. Luzuriaga, D.R. Berry, J.C. Reagan, R.A. Smaldone, J.J. Gassensmith, Biodegradable 3D printed polymer microneedles for transdermal drug delivery, Lab Chip. 18 (2018) 1223–1230. https://doi.org/10.1039/C8LC00098K.

[49]   A. Goyanes, U. Det-Amornrat, J. Wang, A.W. Basit, S. Gaisford, 3D scanning and 3D printing as innovative technologies for fabricating personalized topical drug delivery systems, J. Control. Release. 234 (2016) 41–48. https://doi.org/10.1016/j.jconrel.2016.05.034.

[50]   Z. Muwaffak, A. Goyanes, V. Clark, A.W. Basit, S.T. Hilton, S. Gaisford, Patient-specific 3D scanned and 3D printed antimicrobial polycaprolactone wound dressings, Int. J. Pharm. 527 (2017) 161–170.

https://doi.org/10.1016/j.ijpharm.2017.04.077.

[51]   E. Mathew, J. Domínguez-Robles, S.A. Stewart, E. Mancuso, K. O'Donnell, E. Larrañeta, D.A. Lamprou, Fused Deposition Modeling as an Effective Tool for Anti-Infective Dialysis Catheter Fabrication, ACS Biomater. Sci. Eng. 5 (2019) 6300–6310. https://doi.org/10.1021/acsbiomaterials.9b01185.

[52]   J.A. Weisman, D.H. Ballard, U. Jammalamadaka, K. Tappa, J. Sumerel, H.B. D'Agostino, D.K. Mills, P.K. Woodard, 3D Printed Antibiotic and Chemotherapeutic Eluting Catheters for Potential Use in Interventional Radiology: In Vitro Proof of Concept Study, Acad. Radiol. 26 (2019) 270–274. https://doi.org/10.1016/j.acra.2018.03.022.

[53]   T. Feuerbach, S. Kock, M. Thommes, Slicing parameter optimization for 3D printing of biodegradable drug-eluting tracheal stents, Pharm. Dev. Technol. (2020). https://doi.org/10.1080/10837450.2020.1727921.

[54]   W. Kempin, C. Franz, L.C. Koster, F. Schneider, M. Bogdahn, W. Weitschies, A. Seidlitz, Assessment of different polymers and drug loads for fused deposition modeling of drug loaded implants, Eur. J. Pharm. Biopharm. 115 (2017) 84–93. https://doi.org/10.1016/j.ejpb.2017.02.014.

[55]   S.A. Stewart, J. Domínguez-Robles, V.J. McIlorum, E. Mancuso, D.A. Lamprou, R.F. Donnelly, E. Larrañeta, Development of a biodegradable subcutaneous implant for prolonged drug delivery using 3D printing, Pharmaceutics. 12 (2020) 105. https://doi.org/10.3390/pharmaceutics12020105.

[56]   N. Qamar, N. Abbas, M. Irfan, A. Hussain, M.S. Arshad, S. Latif, F. Mehmood, M.U. Ghori, Personalized 3D printed ciprofloxacin impregnated meshes for the management of hernia, J. Drug Deliv. Sci. Technol. 53 (2019). https://doi.org/10.1016/j.jddst.2019.101164.

[57]   J. Domínguez-Robles, C. Mancinelli, E. Mancuso, I. García-Romero, B.F. Gilmore, L. Casettari, E. Larrañeta, D.A. Lamprou, 3D printing of drug-loaded thermoplastic polyurethane meshes: A potential material for soft tissue reinforcement in vaginal surgery, Pharmaceutics. 12 (2020) 63. https://doi.org/10.3390/pharmaceutics12010063.

[58]   M.A. Wsoo, S. Shahir, S.P. Mohd Bohari, N.H.M. Nayan, S.I.A. Razak, A review on the properties of electrospun cellulose acetate and its application in drug delivery systems: A new perspective, Carbohydr. Res. 491 (2020) 107978. https://doi.org/10.1016/j.carres.2020.107978.

[59]   J. Boetker, J.J. Water, J. Aho, L. Arnfast, A. Bohr, J. Rantanen, Modifying release characteristics from 3D printed drug-eluting products, Eur. J. Pharm. Sci. 90 (2016) 47–52. https://doi.org/10.1016/j.ejps.2016.03.013.

[60]   J. Zhang, X. Feng, H. Patil, R. V. Tiwari, M.A. Repka, Coupling 3D printing with hot-melt extrusion to produce controlled-release tablets, Int. J. Pharm. 519 (2017) 186–197. https://doi.org/10.1016/j.ijpharm.2016.12.049.

[61]   O. Jennotte, N. Koch, A. Lechanteur, B. Evrard, Three-dimensional printing technology as a promising tool in bioavailability enhancement of poorly water-soluble molecules: A review, Int. J. Pharm. 580

(2020) 119200. https://doi.org/10.1016/j.ijpharm.2020.119200.

[62] H. Kadry, T.A. Al-Hilal, A. Keshavarz, F. Alam, C. Xu, A. Joy, F. Ahsan, Multi-purposable filaments of HPMC for 3D printing of medications with tailored drug release and timed-absorption, Int. J. Pharm. 544 (2018) 285–296. https://doi.org/10.1016/j.ijpharm.2018.04.010.

[63] T.C. Okwuosa, D. Stefaniak, B. Arafat, A. Isreb, K.-W.W. Wan, M.A. Alhnan, A Lower Temperature FDM 3D Printing for the Manufacture of Patient-Specific Immediate Release Tablets, Pharm. Res. 33 (2016) 2704–2712. https://doi.org/10.1007/s11095-016-1995-0.

[64] P. Menčík, R. Přikryl, I. Stehnová, V. Melčová, S. Kontárová, S. Figalla, P. Alexy, J. Bočkaj, Effect of selected commercial plasticizers on mechanical, thermal, and morphological properties of poly(3-hydroxybutyrate)/Poly(lactic acid)/plasticizer biodegradable blends for three-dimensional (3D) print, Materials (Basel). 11 (2018). https://doi.org/10.3390/ma11101893.

[65] G. Verreck, The Influence of Plasticizers in Hot-Melt Extrusion, Hot-Melt Extrus. Pharm. Appl. (2012) 93–112. https://doi.org/10.1002/9780470711415.ch5.

[66] M. Elbadawi, Rheological and Mechanical Investigation into the Effect of Different Molecular Weight Poly(ethylene glycol)s on Polycaprolactone-Ciprofloxacin Filaments, ACS Omega. 4 (2019) 5412–5423. https://doi.org/10.1021/acsomega.8b03057.

[67] X. Chai, H. Chai, X. Wang, J. Yang, J. Li, Y. Zhao, W. Cai, T. Tao, X. Xiang, Fused deposition modeling (FDM) 3D printed tablets for intragastric floating delivery of domperidone, Sci. Rep. 7 (2017) 1–9. https://doi.org/10.1038/s41598-017-03097-x.

[68] W. Jamróz, M. Kurek, E. Łyszczarz, J. Szafraniec, J. Knapik-Kowalczuk, K. Syrek, M. Paluch, R. Jachowicz, 3D printed orodispersible films with Aripiprazole, Int. J. Pharm. 533 (2017) 413–420. https://doi.org/10.1016/j.ijpharm.2017.05.052.

[69] T. Ehtezazi, M. Algellay, Y. Islam, M. Roberts, N.M. Dempster, S.D. Sarker, The Application of 3D Printing in the Formulation of Multilayered Fast Dissolving Oral Films, J. Pharm. Sci. 107 (2018) 1076–1085. https://doi.org/10.1016/j.xphs.2017.11.019.

[70] C.I. Gioumouxouzis, O.L. Katsamenis, N. Bouropoulos, D.G. Fatouros, 3D printed oral solid dosage forms containing hydrochlorothiazide for controlled drug delivery, J. Drug Deliv. Sci. Technol. 40 (2017) 164–171. https://doi.org/10.1016/j.jddst.2017.06.008.

[71] A. Melocchi, F. Parietti, G. Loreti, A. Maroni, A. Gazzaniga, L. Zema, 3D printing by fused deposition modeling (FDM) of a swellable/erodible capsular device for oral pulsatile release of drugs, J. Drug Deliv. Sci. Technol. 30 (2015) 360–367. https://doi.org/10.1016/j.jddst.2015.07.016.

[72] T. Tagami, E. Kuwata, N. Sakai, T. Ozeki, Drug incorporation into polymer filament using simple soaking method for tablet preparation using fused deposition modeling, Biol. Pharm. Bull. 42 (2019) 1753–1760. https://doi.org/10.1248/bpb.b19-00482.

[73] G. Verstraete, A. Samaro, W. Grymonpré, V. Vanhoorne, B. Van Snick, M.N. Boone, T. Hellemans, L.

Van Hoorebeke, J.P. Remon, C. Vervaet, 3D printing of high drug loaded dosage forms using thermoplastic polyurethanes, Int. J. Pharm. 536 (2018) 318–325. https://doi.org/10.1016/j.ijpharm.2017.12.002.

[74]   Y. Yang, H. Wang, H. Li, Z. Ou, G. Yang, 3D printed tablets with internal scaffold structure using ethyl cellulose to achieve sustained ibuprofen release, Eur. J. Pharm. Sci. 115 (2018) 11–18. https://doi.org/10.1016/j.ejps.2018.01.005.

[75]   R.C.R. Beck, P.S. Chaves, A. Goyanes, B. Vukosavljevic, A. Buanz, M. Windbergs, A.W. Basit, S. Gaisford, 3D printed tablets loaded with polymeric nanocapsules: An innovative approach to produce customized drug delivery systems, Int. J. Pharm. 528 (2017) 268–279. https://doi.org/10.1016/j.ijpharm.2017.05.074.

[76]   M. Sadia, A. Isreb, I. Abbadi, M. Isreb, D. Aziz, A. Selo, P. Timmins, M.A. Alhnan, From 'fixed dose combinations' to 'a dynamic dose combiner': 3D printed bi-layer antihypertensive tablets, Eur. J. Pharm. Sci. 123 (2018) 484–494. https://doi.org/10.1016/j.ejps.2018.07.045.

[77]   H.E. Gültekin, S. Tort, F. Acartürk, An Effective Technology for the Development of Immediate Release Solid Dosage Forms Containing Low-Dose Drug: Fused Deposition Modeling 3D Printing, Pharm. Res. 36 (2019). https://doi.org/10.1007/s11095-019-2655-y.

[78]   M. Alhijjaj, P. Belton, S. Qi, An investigation into the use of polymer blends to improve the printability of and regulate drug release from pharmaceutical solid dispersions prepared via fused deposition modeling (FDM) 3D printing, Eur. J. Pharm. Biopharm. 108 (2016) 111–125. https://doi.org/10.1016/j.ejpb.2016.08.016.

[79]   C.I. Gioumouxouzis, A. Baklavaridis, O.L. Katsamenis, C.K. Markopoulou, N. Bouropoulos, D. Tzetzis, D.G. Fatouros, A 3D printed bilayer oral solid dosage form combining metformin for prolonged and glimepiride for immediate drug delivery, Eur. J. Pharm. Sci. 120 (2018) 40–52. https://doi.org/10.1016/j.ejps.2018.04.020.

[80]   B. Arafat, M. Wojsz, A. Isreb, R.T. Forbes, M. Isreb, W. Ahmed, T. Arafat, M.A. Alhnan, Tablet fragmentation without a disintegrant: A novel design approach for accelerating disintegration and drug release from 3D printed cellulosic tablets, Eur. J. Pharm. Sci. 118 (2018) 191–199. https://doi.org/10.1016/j.ejps.2018.03.019.

[81]   H. Öblom, J. Zhang, M. Pimparade, I. Speer, M. Preis, M. Repka, N. Sandler, 3D-Printed Isoniazid Tablets for the Treatment and Prevention of Tuberculosis—Personalized Dosing and Drug Release, AAPS PharmSciTech. 20 (2019). https://doi.org/10.1208/s12249-018-1233-7.

[82]   J. Zhang, W. Yang, A.Q. Vo, X. Feng, X. Ye, D.W. Kim, M.A. Repka, Hydroxypropyl methylcellulose-based controlled release dosage by melt extrusion and 3D printing: Structure and drug release correlation, Carbohydr. Polym. 177 (2017) 49–57. https://doi.org/10.1016/j.carbpol.2017.08.058.

[83]   A. Goyanes, F. Fina, A. Martorana, D. Sedough, S. Gaisford, A.W. Basit, Development of modified release 3D printed tablets (printlets) with pharmaceutical excipients using additive manufacturing, Int. J.

Pharm. Accepted (2017) 21–30. https://doi.org/10.1016/j.ijpharm.2017.05.021.

[84]   G. Kollamaram, D.M. Croker, G.M. Walker, A. Goyanes, A.W. Basit, S. Gaisford, Low temperature fused deposition modeling (FDM) 3D printing of thermolabile drugs, Int. J. Pharm. 545 (2018) 144–152. https://doi.org/10.1016/j.ijpharm.2018.04.055.

[85]   J.J. Water, A. Bohr, J. Boetker, J. Aho, N. Sandler, H.M.M. Nielsen, J. Rantanen, Three-dimensional printing of drug-eluting implants: Preparation of an antimicrobial polylactide feedstock material, J. Pharm. Sci. 104 (2015) 1099–1107. https://doi.org/10.1002/jps.24305.

[86]   A. Isreb, K. Baj, M. Wojsz, M. Isreb, M. Peak, M.A. Alhnan, 3D printed oral theophylline doses with innovative 'radiator-like' design: Impact of polyethylene oxide (PEO) molecular weight, Int. J. Pharm. 564 (2019) 98–105. https://doi.org/10.1016/j.ijpharm.2019.04.017.

[87]   A. Goyanes, J. Wang, A. Buanz, R. Martínez-Pacheco, R. Telford, S. Gaisford, A.W. Basit, 3D Printing of Medicines: Engineering Novel Oral Devices with Unique Design and Drug Release Characteristics, Mol. Pharm. 12 (2015) 4077–4084. https://doi.org/10.1021/acs.molpharmaceut.5b00510.

[88]   A. Goyanes, M. Kobayashi, R. Martínez-pacheco, S. Gaisford, A.W. Basit, Fused- filament 3D printing of drug products: Microstructure analysis and drug release characteristics of PVA-based caplets, Int. J. Pharm. 514 (2016) 290–295. https://doi.org/10.1016/j.ijpharm.2016.06.021.

[89]   T. Tagami, N. Nagata, N. Hayashi, E. Ogawa, K. Fukushige, N. Sakai, T. Ozeki, Defined drug release from 3D-printed composite tablets consisting of drug-loaded polyvinylalcohol and a water-soluble or water-insoluble polymer filler, Int. J. Pharm. 543 (2018) 361–367. https://doi.org/10.1016/j.ijpharm.2018.03.057.

[90]   T.C. Okwuosa, B.C. Pereira, B. Arafat, M. Cieszynska, A. Isreb, M.A. Alhnan, Fabricating a Shell-Core Delayed Release Tablet Using Dual FDM 3D Printing for Patient-Centred Therapy, Pharm. Res. 34 (2017) 427–437. https://doi.org/10.1007/s11095-016-2073-3.

[91]   I. Major, S. Lastakchi, M. Dalton, C. McConville, Implantable drug delivery systems, in: Eng. Drug Deliv. Syst., Elsevier, 2020: pp. 111–146. https://doi.org/10.1016/B978-0-08-102548-2.00005-6.

[92]   L.W. Kleiner, J.C. Wright, Y. Wang, Evolution of implantable and insertable drug delivery systems, J. Control. Release. 181 (2014) 1–10. https://doi.org/10.1016/j.jconrel.2014.02.006.

[93]   S.A. Stewart, J. Domínguez-Robles, R.F. Donnelly, E. Larrañeta, Implantable polymeric drug delivery devices: Classification, manufacture, materials, and clinical applications, Polymers (Basel). 10 (2018). https://doi.org/10.3390/polym10121379.

[94]   A. Kumar, J. Pillai, Implantable drug delivery systems: An overview, in: Nanostructures Eng. Cells, Tissues Organs From Des. to Appl., Elsevier, 2018: pp. 473–511. https://doi.org/10.1016/B978-0-12-813665-2.00013-2.

[95]   C. Schneider, R. Langer, D. Loveday, D. Hair, Applications of ethylene vinyl acetate copolymers (EVA) in drug delivery systems, J. Control. Release. 262 (2017) 284–295.

https://doi.org/10.1016/j.jconrel.2017.08.004.

[96]   Y. Fu, W.J. Kao, Drug release kinetics and transport mechanisms of non-degradable and degradable polymeric delivery systems, Expert Opin. Drug Deliv. 7 (2010) 429–444. https://doi.org/10.1517/17425241003602259.

[97]   A. Mane, N. Maheshwari, P. Ghode, M.C. Sharma, R.K. Tekade, Approaches to the Development of Implantable Therapeutic Systems, in: Biomater. Bionanotechnol., Elsevier, 2019: pp. 191–224. https://doi.org/10.1016/B978-0-12-814427-5.00006-8.

[98]   M.B. Lowinger, S.E. Barrett, F. Zhang, R.O. Williams, Sustained release drug delivery applications of polyurethanes, Pharmaceutics. 10 (2018) 55. https://doi.org/10.3390/pharmaceutics10020055.

[99]   D.N. Kapoor, A. Bhatia, R. Kaur, R. Sharma, G. Kaur, S. Dhawan, PLGA: a unique polymer for drug delivery, Ther. Deliv. 6 (2015) 41–58. https://doi.org/10.4155/tde.14.91.

[100]   R. Song, M. Murphy, C. Li, K. Ting, C. Soo, Z. Zheng, Current development of biodegradable polymeric materials for biomedical applications, Drug Des. Devel. Ther. Volume 12 (2018) 3117–3145. https://doi.org/10.2147/DDDT.S165440.

[101]   J.A.D. Sequeira, A.C. Santos, J. Serra, F. Veiga, A.J. Ribeiro, Poly(lactic-co-glycolic acid) (PLGA) matrix implants, in: Nanostructures Eng. Cells, Tissues Organs From Des. to Appl., Elsevier, 2018: pp. 375–402. https://doi.org/10.1016/B978-0-12-813665-2.00010-7.

[102]   P.W. Lee, J.K. Pokorski, Poly(lactic-co-glycolic acid) devices: Production and applications for sustained protein delivery, Wiley Interdiscip. Rev. Nanomedicine Nanobiotechnology. 10 (2018) e1516. https://doi.org/10.1002/wnan.1516.

[103]   C. Bode, H. Kranz, A. Fivez, F. Siepmann, J. Siepmann, Often neglected: PLGA/PLA swelling orchestrates drug release: HME implants, J. Control. Release. 306 (2019) 97–107. https://doi.org/10.1016/j.jconrel.2019.05.039.

[104]   V. Karavelidis, E. Karavas, D. Giliopoulos, S. Papadimitriou, D. Bikiaris, Evaluating the effects of crystallinity in new biocompatible polyester nanocarriers on drug release behavior, Int. J. Nanomedicine. 6 (2011) 3021. https://doi.org/10.2147/ijn.s26016.

[105]   N. Kamaly, B. Yameen, J. Wu, O.C. Farokhzad, Degradable controlled-release polymers and polymeric nanoparticles: Mechanisms of controlling drug release, Chem. Rev. 116 (2016) 2602–2663. https://doi.org/10.1021/acs.chemrev.5b00346.

[106]   S. Sonam, H. Chaudhary, V. Arora, K. Kholi, V. Kumar, Effect of physicochemical properties of biodegradable polymers on nano drug delivery, Polym. Rev. 53 (2013) 546–567. https://doi.org/10.1080/15583724.2013.828751.

[107]   X. Huang, C.S. Brazel, Analysis of burst release of proxyphylline from poly(vinyl alcohol) hydrogels, Chem. Eng. Commun. 190 (2003) 519–532. https://doi.org/10.1080/00986440302081.

[108]   J.A.D. Sequeira, A.C. Santos, J. Serra, C. Estevens, R. Seiça, F. Veiga, A.J. Ribeiro, Subcutaneous delivery of biotherapeutics: challenges at the injection site, Expert Opin. Drug Deliv. 16 (2019) 143–151. https://doi.org/10.1080/17425247.2019.1568408.

[109]   S. Fredenberg, M. Wahlgren, M. Reslow, A. Axelsson, The mechanisms of drug release in poly(lactic-co-glycolic acid)-based drug delivery systems--a review., Int. J. Pharm. 415 (2011) 34–52. https://doi.org/10.1016/j.ijpharm.2011.05.049.

[110]   B. Sun, M. Zhang, J. Shen, Z. He, P. Fatehi, Y. Ni, Applications of Cellulose-based Materials in Sustained Drug Delivery Systems, Curr. Med. Chem. 26 (2018) 2485–2501. https://doi.org/10.2174/0929867324666170705143308.

[111]   K. Löbmann, A.J. Svagan, Cellulose nanofibers as excipient for the delivery of poorly soluble drugs, Int. J. Pharm. 533 (2017) 285–297. https://doi.org/10.1016/j.ijpharm.2017.09.064.

[112]   Z. Guo, D. Bo, Y. He, X. Luo, H. Li, Degradation properties of chitosan microspheres/poly(L-lactic acid) composite in vitro and in vivo, Carbohydr. Polym. 193 (2018) 1–8. https://doi.org/10.1016/j.carbpol.2018.03.067.

[113]   J. Gao, Y. Xu, Y. Zheng, X. Wang, S. Li, G. Yan, J. Wang, R. Tang, pH-sensitive carboxymethyl chitosan hydrogels via acid-labile ortho ester linkage as an implantable drug delivery system, Carbohydr. Polym. 225 (2019) 115237. https://doi.org/10.1016/j.carbpol.2019.115237.

[114]   U. Garg, S. Chauhan, U. Nagaich, N. Jain, Current advances in chitosan nanoparticles based drug delivery and targeting, Adv. Pharm. Bull. 9 (2019) 195–204. https://doi.org/10.15171/apb.2019.023.

[115]   T. Yucel, M.L. Lovett, D.L. Kaplan, Silk-based biomaterials for sustained drug delivery, J. Control. Release. 190 (2014) 381–397. https://doi.org/10.1016/j.jconrel.2014.05.059.

[116]   K.E. Washington, R.N. Kularatne, V. Karmegam, M.C. Biewer, M.C. Stefan, Recent advances in aliphatic polyesters for drug delivery applications, Wiley Interdiscip. Rev. Nanomedicine Nanobiotechnology. 9 (2017) e1446. https://doi.org/10.1002/wnan.1446.

[117]   O.A. Abu-Diak, G.P. Andrews, D.S. Jones, Hydrophobic polymers of pharmaceutical significance, in: Fundam. Appl. Control. Release Drug Deliv., Springer US, 2012: pp. 47–73. https://doi.org/10.1007/978-1-4614-0881-9_3.

[118]   K. Mäder, E. Lehner, A. Liebau, S.K. Plontke, Controlled drug release to the inner ear: Concepts, materials, mechanisms, and performance, Hear. Res. 368 (2018) 49–66. https://doi.org/10.1016/j.heares.2018.03.006.

[119]   J.H. Park, M. Ye, K. Park, Biodegradable polymers for microencapsulation of drugs, Molecules. 10 (2005) 146–161. https://doi.org/10.3390/10010146.

[120]   R.A. Siegel, M.J. Rathbone, Overview of controlled release mechanisms, in: Fundam. Appl. Control. Release Drug Deliv., Springer US, 2012: pp. 19–43. https://doi.org/10.1007/978-1-4614-0881-9_2.

[121] R.P. Brannigan, A.P. Dove, Synthesis, properties and biomedical applications of hydrolytically degradable materials based on aliphatic polyesters and polycarbonates, Biomater. Sci. 5 (2016) 9. https://doi.org/10.1039/c6bm00584e.

[122] H.K. Makadia, S.J. Siegel, Poly Lactic-co-Glycolic Acid (PLGA) as biodegradable controlled drug delivery carrier, Polymers (Basel). 3 (2011) 1377–1397. https://doi.org/10.3390/polym3031377.

[123] S.L. Fialho, A. Da, S. Cunha, A. Da Silva Cunha, Manufacturing techniques of biodegradable implants intended for intraocular application, Drug Deliv. J. Deliv. Target. Ther. Agents. 12 (2005) 109–116. https://doi.org/10.1080/10717540590921432.

[124] X. Zhao, D. Hobson, Z.Y.W. Lin, W. Cuia, Electrospun biodegradable polyester micro-/nanofibers for drug delivery and their clinical applications, in: Handb. Polyest. Drug Deliv. Syst., Hardcover, 2016: pp. 125–158. https://doi.org/10.4032/9789814669665.

[125] M.S. Islam, B.C. Ang, A. Andriyana, A.M. Afifi, A review on fabrication of nanofibers via electrospinning and their applications, SN Appl. Sci. 1 (2019) 1–16. https://doi.org/10.1007/s42452-019-1288-4.

[126] D.K. Tan, M. Maniruzzaman, A. Nokhodchi, Advanced pharmaceutical applications of hot-melt extrusion coupled with fused deposition modelling (FDM) 3D printing for personalised drug delivery, MDPI AG, 2018. https://doi.org/10.3390/pharmaceutics10040203.

[127] P.W. Lee, S. Shukla, J.D. Wallat, C. Danda, N.F. Steinmetz, J. Maia, J.K. Pokorski, Biodegradable Viral Nanoparticle/Polymer Implants Prepared via Melt-Processing, ACS Nano. 11 (2017) 8777–8789. https://doi.org/10.1021/acsnano.7b02786.

[128] L. Duque, M. Körber, R. Bodmeier, Improving release completeness from PLGA-based implants for the acid-labile model protein ovalbumin, Int. J. Pharm. 538 (2018) 139–146. https://doi.org/10.1016/j.ijpharm.2018.01.026.

[129] A. Cossé, C. König, A. Lamprecht, K.G. Wagner, Hot Melt Extrusion for Sustained Protein Release: Matrix Erosion and In Vitro Release of PLGA-Based Implants, AAPS PharmSciTech. (2016). https://doi.org/10.1208/s12249-016-0548-5.

[130] Z. Ghalanbor, M. Körber, R. Bodmeier, Protein release from poly(lactide-co-glycolide) implants prepared by hot-melt extrusion: Thioester formation as a reason for incomplete release, Int. J. Pharm. 438 (2012) 302–306. https://doi.org/10.1016/j.ijpharm.2012.09.015.

[131] A.J. Pollard, E.M. Bijker, A guide to vaccinology: from basic principles to new developments, Nat. Rev. Immunol. 21 (2021) 83–100. https://doi.org/10.1038/s41577-020-00479-7.

[132] W. Wang, S. Singh, D.L. Zeng, K. King, S. Nema, Antibody structure, instability, and formulation, J. Pharm. Sci. 96 (2007) 1–26. https://doi.org/10.1002/jps.20727.

[133] S. Awwad, U. Angkawinitwong, Overview of Antibody Drug Delivery, Pharmaceutics. 10 (2018) 83. https://doi.org/10.3390/pharmaceutics10030083.

[134] N.A.P.S. Buss, S.J. Henderson, M. McFarlane, J.M. Shenton, L. De Haan, Monoclonal antibody therapeutics: History and future, Curr. Opin. Pharmacol. 12 (2012) 615–622. https://doi.org/10.1016/j.coph.2012.08.001.

[135] S. Boune, P. Hu, A.L. Epstein, L.A. Khawli, Principles of N-Linked Glycosylation Variations of IgG-Based Therapeutics: Pharmacokinetic and Functional Considerations, Antibodies. 9 (2020) 22. https://doi.org/10.3390/antib9020022.

[136] R.J. Sola, K. Griebenow, Effects of glycosylate on the stability of protein pharmaceuticals, J. Pharm. Sci. 98 (2009) 1223–1245. https://doi.org/10.1002/jps.21504.

[137] R. Wada, M. Matsui, N. Kawasaki, Influence of N-glycosylation on effector functions and thermal stability of glycoengineered IgG1 monoclonal antibody with homogeneous glycoforms, MAbs. 11 (2019) 350–372. https://doi.org/10.1080/19420862.2018.1551044.

[138] V.M. Balcão, M.M.D.C. Vila, Structural and functional stabilization of protein entities: State-of-the-art, Adv. Drug Deliv. Rev. 93 (2015) 25–41. https://doi.org/10.1016/j.addr.2014.10.005.

[139] M.C. Manning, D.K. Chou, B.M. Murphy, R.W. Payne, D.S. Katayama, Stability of protein pharmaceuticals: An update, Pharm. Res. 27 (2010) 544–575. https://doi.org/10.1007/s11095-009-0045-6.

[140] Y. Le Basle, P. Chennell, N. Tokhadze, A. Astier, V. Sautou, Physicochemical Stability of Monoclonal Antibodies: A Review, J. Pharm. Sci. 109 (2020) 169–190. https://doi.org/10.1016/j.xphs.2019.08.009.

[141] J. Horn, H. Mahler, W. Friess, Drying for Stabilization of Protein Formulations, in: Dry. Technol. Biotechnol. Pharm. Appl., Wiley, 2020: pp. 91–119. https://doi.org/10.1002/9783527802104.ch4.

[142] D. Gervais, Protein deamidation in biopharmaceutical manufacture: Understanding, control and impact, J. Chem. Technol. Biotechnol. 91 (2016) 569–575. https://doi.org/10.1002/jctb.4850.

[143] L. Jia, Y. Sun, Protein asparagine deamidation prediction based on structures with machine learning methods, PLoS One. 12 (2017). https://doi.org/10.1371/journal.pone.0181347.

[144] E.M. Topp, L. Zhang, H. Zhao, R.W. Payne, G.J. Evans, M.C. Manning, Chemical Instability in Peptide and Protein Pharmaceuticals, in: Formul. Process Dev. Strateg. Manuf. Biopharm., John Wiley & Sons, Inc., Hoboken, NJ, USA, 2010: pp. 41–67. https://doi.org/10.1002/9780470595886.ch2.

[145] M.E. Krause, E. Sahin, Chemical and physical instabilities in manufacturing and storage of therapeutic proteins, Curr. Opin. Biotechnol. 60 (2019) 159–167. https://doi.org/10.1016/j.copbio.2019.01.014.

[146] M.L.L. Houchin, E.M.M. Topp, Chemical Degradation of Peptides and Proteins in PLGA: A Review of Reactions and Mechanisms, J. Pharm. Sci. 97 (2008) 2395–2404. https://doi.org/10.1002/jps.21176.

[147] M. Shirangi, W.E. Hennink, G.W. Somsen, C.F. Van Nostrum, Acylation of arginine in goserelin-loaded PLGA microspheres, Eur. J. Pharm. Biopharm. 99 (2016) 18–23. https://doi.org/10.1016/j.ejpb.2015.11.008.

[148] S. Kharel, A. Gautam, A. Dickescheid, S.C.J. Loo, Hollow Microparticles as a Superior Delivery System over Solid Microparticles for the Encapsulation of Peptides, Pharm. Res. 35 (2018) 185–195. https://doi.org/10.1007/s11095-018-2461-y.

[149] J. Liu, Y. Xu, Y. Wang, H. Ren, Z. Meng, K. Liu, Z. Liu, H. Huang, X. Li, Effect of inner pH on peptide acylation within PLGA microspheres, Eur. J. Pharm. Sci. 134 (2019) 69–80. https://doi.org/10.1016/j.ejps.2019.04.017.

[150] W. Wang, C.J. Roberts, Protein aggregation – Mechanisms, detection, and control, Int. J. Pharm. 550 (2018) 251–268. https://doi.org/10.1016/j.ijpharm.2018.08.043.

[151] C. Quan, E. Alcala, I. Petkovska, D. Matthews, E. Canova-Davis, R. Taticek, S. Ma, A study in glycation of a therapeutic recombinant humanized monoclonal antibody: Where it is, how it got there, and how it affects charge-based behavior, Anal. Biochem. 373 (2008) 179–191. https://doi.org/10.1016/j.ab.2007.09.027.

[152] S. Ravuluri, R. Bansal, N. Chhabra, A.S. Rathore, Kinetics and Characterization of Non-enzymatic Fragmentation of Monoclonal Antibody Therapeutics, Pharm. Res. 35 (2018). https://doi.org/10.1007/s11095-018-2415-4.

[153] J. Vlasak, R. Ionescu, Fragmentation of monoclonal antibodies, MAbs. 3 (2011) 253–263. https://doi.org/10.4161/mabs.3.3.15608.

[154] B. Huang, S. Singamneni, Raster angle mechanics in fused deposition modelling, J. Compos. Mater. 0 (2014) 1–21. https://doi.org/10.1177/0021998313519153.

[155] M.A. Mensink, H.W. Frijlink, K. van der Voort Maarschalk, W.L.J. Hinrichs, How sugars protect proteins in the solid state and during drying (review): Mechanisms of stabilization in relation to stress conditions, Eur. J. Pharm. Biopharm. 114 (2017) 288–295. https://doi.org/10.1016/j.ejpb.2017.01.024.

[156] L. (Lucy) L. Chang, M.J. Pikal, Mechanisms of protein stabilization in the solid state, Elsevier, 2009. https://doi.org/10.1002/jps.21825.

[157] C.J. Roberts, Therapeutic protein aggregation: Mechanisms, design, and control, Trends Biotechnol. 32 (2014) 372–380. https://doi.org/10.1016/j.tibtech.2014.05.005.

[158] U. Angkawinitwong, G. Sharma, P.T. Khaw, S. Brocchini, G.R. Williams, Solid-state protein formulations, Ther. Deliv. 6 (2015) 59–82. https://doi.org/10.4155/tde.14.98.

[159] W. Wang, Protein aggregation and its inhibition in biopharmaceutics, Int. J. Pharm. 289 (2005) 1–30. https://doi.org/10.1016/j.ijpharm.2004.11.014.

[160] W. Li, P. Prabakaran, W. Chen, Z. Zhu, Y. Feng, D. Dimitrov, Antibody Aggregation: Insights from Sequence and Structure, Antibodies. 5 (2016) 19. https://doi.org/10.3390/antib5030019.

[161] F. Emami, A. Vatanara, E.J. Park, D.H. Na, Drying technologies for the stability and bioavailability of biopharmaceuticals, Pharmaceutics. 10 (2018). https://doi.org/10.3390/pharmaceutics10030131.

[162] A. Ziaee, A.B. Albadarin, L. Padrela, T. Femmer, E. O'Reilly, G. Walker, Spray drying of pharmaceuticals and biopharmaceuticals: Critical parameters and experimental process optimization approaches, Eur. J. Pharm. Sci. 127 (2019) 300–318. https://doi.org/10.1016/j.ejps.2018.10.026.

[163] G.A. Ledet, R.A. Graves, L.A. Bostanian, T.K. Mandal, Spray-Drying of Biopharmaceuticals, in: Lyophilized Biol. Vaccines, Springer New York, 2015: pp. 273–297. https://doi.org/10.1007/978-1-4939-2383-0_12.

[164] R.H. Walters, B. Bhatnagar, S. Tchessalov, K.I. Izutsu, K. Tsumoto, S. Ohtake, Next generation drying technologies for pharmaceutical applications, J. Pharm. Sci. 103 (2014) 2673–2695. https://doi.org/10.1002/jps.23998.

[165] W.F. Tonnis, M.A. Mensink, A. De Jager, K. Van Der Voort Maarschalk, H.W. Frijlink, W.L.J. Hinrichs, Size and molecular flexibility of sugars determine the storage stability of freeze-dried proteins, Mol. Pharm. 12 (2015) 684–694. https://doi.org/10.1021/mp500423z.

[166] F. Depreter, G. Pilcer, K. Amighi, Inhaled proteins: Challenges and perspectives, Int. J. Pharm. 447 (2013) 251–280. https://doi.org/10.1016/j.ijpharm.2013.02.031.

[167] S. Mangal, F. Meiser, G. Tan, T. Gengenbach, J. Denman, M.R. Rowles, I. Larson, D.A.V. Morton, Relationship between surface concentration of l-leucine and bulk powder properties in spray dried formulations, Eur. J. Pharm. Biopharm. 94 (2015) 160–169. https://doi.org/10.1016/j.ejpb.2015.04.035.

[168] D.M. Piedmonte, A. Hair, P. Baker, L. Brych, K. Nagapudi, H. Lin, W. Cao, S. Hershenson, G. Ratnaswamy, Sorbitol crystallization-induced aggregation in frozen mAb formulations, J. Pharm. Sci. 104 (2015) 686–697. https://doi.org/10.1002/jps.24141.

[169] R. Vaishya, V. Khurana, S. Patel, A.K. Mitra, Long-term delivery of protein therapeutics, Expert Opin. Drug Deliv. 12 (2015) 415–440. https://doi.org/10.1517/17425247.2015.961420.

[170] S. Marquette, C. Peerboom, A. Yates, L. Denis, J. Goole, K. Amighi, Encapsulation of immunoglobulin G by solid-in-oil-in-water: Effect of process parameters on microsphere properties, Eur. J. Pharm. Biopharm. 86 (2014) 393–403. https://doi.org/10.1016/j.ejpb.2013.10.013.

[171] T.R. Hoare, D.S. Kohane, Hydrogels in drug delivery: Progress and challenges, Polymer (Guildf). 49 (2008) 1993–2007. https://doi.org/10.1016/j.polymer.2008.01.027.

[172] A. Arrighi, S. Marquette, C. Peerboom, L. Denis, J. Goole, K. Amighi, Development of PLGA microparticles with high immunoglobulin G-loaded levels and sustained-release properties obtained by spray-drying a water-in-oil emulsion, Int. J. Pharm. 566 (2019) 291–298. https://doi.org/10.1016/j.ijpharm.2019.05.070.

[173] M. Batens, J. Massant, B. Teodorescu, G. Van den Mooter, Formulating monoclonal antibodies as powders for reconstitution at high concentration using spray drying: Models and pitfalls, Eur. J. Pharm. Biopharm. 127 (2018) 407–422. https://doi.org/10.1016/j.ejpb.2018.02.002.

[174] M. Baiardo, G. Frisoni, M. Scandola, M. Rimelen, D. Lips, K. Ruffieux, E. Wintermantel, Thermal and

mechanical properties of plasticized poly(L-lactic acid), J. Appl. Polym. Sci. 90 (2003) 1731–1738. https://doi.org/10.1002/app.12549.

[175] J. Cantrell, S. Rohde, D. Damiani, R. Gurnani, L. Disandro, J. Anton, A. Young, A. Jerez, D. Steinbach, C. Kroese, P. Ifju, Experimental Characterization of the Mechanical Properties of 3D-Printed ABS and Polycarbonate Parts, Univ. Florida. (2011) 89–105. https://doi.org/10.1007/978-3-319-41600-7_11.

[176] J. Kotlinski, Mechanical properties of commercial rapid prototyping materials, Rapid Prototyp. J. 20 (2014) 499–510. https://doi.org/10.1108/RPJ-06-2012-0052.

[177] ASTM, ASTM D638 – 14. Standard Test Method for Tensile Properties of Plastics, Annu. B. ASTM Stand. (2014) 1–20. https://doi.org/10.1520/D0638-14.

[178] T. Scientific, Pierce ® BCA Protein Assay Kit, 2011. https://doi.org/10.1016/j.ijproman.2010.02.012.

[179] Y. Song, Y. Li, W. Song, K. Yee, K.Y. Lee, V.L. Tagarielli, Measurements of the mechanical response of unidirectional 3D-printed PLA, Mater. Des. 123 (2017) 154–164. https://doi.org/10.1016/j.matdes.2017.03.051.

[180] S. Farah, D.G. Anderson, R. Langer, Physical and mechanical properties of PLA, and their functions in widespread applications - A comprehensive review, Adv. Drug Deliv. Rev. 107 (2016) 367–392. https://doi.org/10.1016/j.addr.2016.06.012.

[181] J.A. Morais, Mr. Lobato, The New EMEA Guideline on the Investigation of Bioequivalence, Rev. Port. Farmacoter. Vol. 1 (2009) 76–80. https://www.ema.europa.eu/en/documents/scientific-guideline/guideline-investigation-bioequivalence-rev1_en.pdf (accessed September 1, 2020).

[182] V.P. Shah, Y. Tsong, P. Sathe, J.P. Liu, In vitro dissolution profile comparison- Statistics and analysis of the similarity factor, f2, Pharm. Res. 15 (1998) 889–896. https://doi.org/10.1023/A:1011976615750.

[183] L. Xiao, B. Wang, G. Yang, M. Gauthier, Poly (Lactic Acid) -Based Biomaterials : Synthesis , Modification and Applications, Iomedical Sci. Eng. Technol. (2012) 249–283. https://doi.org/10.5772/23927.

[184] H. Patil, R. V. Tiwari, M.A. Repka, Hot-Melt Extrusion: from Theory to Application in Pharmaceutical Formulation, AAPS PharmSciTech. 17 (2015) 20–42. https://doi.org/10.1208/s12249-015-0360-7.

[185] M.P. Arrieta, M.D.M. Castro-López, E. Rayón, L.F. Barral-Losada, J.M. López-Vilariño, J. López, M.V. González-Rodríguez, Plasticized poly(lactic acid)-poly(hydroxybutyrate) (PLA-PHB) blends incorporated with catechin intended for active food-packaging applications, J. Agric. Food Chem. 62 (2014) 10170–10180. https://doi.org/10.1021/jf5029812.

[186] European Medicines Agency (EMA), ICH guideline Q3C (R6) on impurities: Guideline for Residual Solvents, Int. Conf. Harmon. Tech. Requir. Regist. Pharm. Hum. Use. 31 (2019) 24. www.ema.europa.eu/contactsTelephone+31 (accessed April 3, 2021).

[187] R. Jani, D. Patel, Hot melt extrusion: An industrially feasible approach for casting orodispersible film,

Asian J. Pharm. Sci. 10 (2014) 292–305. https://doi.org/10.1016/j.ajps.2015.03.002.

[188] M. Maiza, M.T. Benaniba, G. Quintard, V. Massardier-Nageotte, Biobased additive plasticizing Polylactic acid (PLA), Polimeros. 25 (2015) 581–590. https://doi.org/10.1590/0104-1428.1986.

[189] O. Martin, L. Avérous, Poly(lactic acid): Plasticization and properties of biodegradable multiphase systems, Polymer (Guildf). 42 (2001) 6209–6219. https://doi.org/10.1016/S0032-3861(01)00086-6.

[190] A. Greco, F. Ferrari, A. Maffezzoli, Thermal analysis of poly(lactic acid) plasticized by cardanol derivatives, J. Therm. Anal. Calorim. (2018) 1–7. https://doi.org/10.1007/s10973-018-7059-4.

[191] Y. Wang, Y. Qin, Y. Zhang, M. Yuan, H. Li, M. Yuan, Effects of N-octyl lactate as plasticizer on the thermal and functional properties of extruded PLA-based films, Int. J. Biol. Macromol. 67 (2014) 58–63. https://doi.org/10.1016/j.ijbiomac.2014.02.048.

[192] S. Fehri, P. Cinelli, M.-B. Coltelli, I. Anguillesi, A. Lazzeri, Thermal Properties of Plasticized Poly (Lactic Acid) (PLA) Containing Nucleating Agent, Int. J. Chem. Eng. Appl. 7 (2016) 85–88. https://doi.org/10.7763/IJCEA.2016.V7.548.

[193] D. Li, Y. Jiang, S. Lv, X. Liu, J. Gu, Q. Chen, Y. Zhang, Preparation of plasticized poly (lactic acid) and its influence on the properties of composite materials, PLoS One. 13 (2018) 1–15. https://doi.org/10.1371/journal.pone.0193520.

[194] E. Fuenmayor, M. Forde, A. V. Healy, D.M. Devine, J.G. Lyons, C. McConville, I. Major, Material considerations for fused-filament fabrication of solid dosage forms, Pharmaceutics. 10 (2018) 44. https://doi.org/10.3390/pharmaceutics10020044.

[195] S. Wang, L. Capoen, D.R. D'hooge, L. Cardon, Can the melt flow index be used to predict the success of fused deposition modelling of commercial poly(lactic acid) filaments into 3D printed materials?, Plast. Rubber Compos. 47 (2018) 9–16. https://doi.org/10.1080/14658011.2017.1397308.

[196] J. Torres, M. Cole, A. Owji, Z. DeMastry, A.P. Gordon, An approach for mechanical property optimization of fused deposition modeling with polylactic acid via design of experiments, Rapid Prototyp. J. 22 (2016) 387–404. https://doi.org/10.1108/RPJ-07-2014-0083.

[197] O.S. Carneiro, A.F. Silva, R. Gomes, Fused deposition modeling with polypropylene, Mater. Des. 83 (2015) 768–776. https://doi.org/10.1016/j.matdes.2015.06.053.

[198] J. Chacón, M. Caminero, E. García-Plaza, P. Núñez, Additive manufacturing of PLA structures using fused deposition modelling: effect of process parameters on mechanical properties and their optimal selection, Mater. Des. 124 (2017) 143–157. https://doi.org/10.1016/j.matdes.2017.03.065.

[199] M.A. Abdelwahab, A. Flynn, B. Sen Chiou, S. Imam, W. Orts, E. Chiellini, Thermal, mechanical and morphological characterization of plasticized PLA-PHB blends, Polym. Degrad. Stab. 97 (2012) 1822–1828. https://doi.org/10.1016/j.polymdegradstab.2012.05.036.

[200] A. Södergård, M. Stolt, Properties of lactic acid based polymers and their correlation with composition,

Prog. Polym. Sci. 27 (2002) 1123–1163. https://doi.org/10.1016/S0079-6700(02)00012-6.

[201]   Y. Jin, Y. Wan, B. Zhang, Z. Liu, Modeling of the chemical finishing process for polylactic acid parts in fused deposition modeling and investigation of its tensile properties, J. Mater. Process. Technol. 240 (2017) 233–239. https://doi.org/10.1016/j.jmatprotec.2016.10.003.

[202]   B.M. Tymrak, M. Kreiger, J.M. Pearce, Mechanical properties of components fabricated with open-source 3-D printers under realistic environmental conditions, Mater. Des. 58 (2014) 242–246. https://doi.org/10.1016/j.matdes.2014.02.038.

[203]   K.G.J. Christiyan, U. Chandrasekhar, K. Venkateswarlu, A study on the influence of process parameters on the Mechanical Properties of 3D printed ABS composite, IOP Conf. Ser. Mater. Sci. Eng. 114 (2016) 012109. https://doi.org/10.1088/1757-899X/114/1/012109.

[204]   S. Wasti, S. Adhikari, Use of Biomaterials for 3D Printing by Fused Deposition Modeling Technique: A Review, Front. Chem. 8 (2020) 315. https://doi.org/10.3389/fchem.2020.00315.

[205]   M. Kariz, M. Sernek, M. Obućina, M.K. Kuzman, Effect of wood content in FDM filament on properties of 3D printed parts, Mater. Today Commun. 14 (2018) 135–140. https://doi.org/10.1016/j.mtcomm.2017.12.016.

[206]   Z. Ghalanbor, M. Körber, R. Bodmeier, Improved lysozyme stability and release properties of Poly(lactide-co- glycolide) implants prepared by hot-melt extrusion, Pharm. Res. 27 (2010) 371–379. https://doi.org/10.1007/s11095-009-0033-x.

[207]   J. Aho, J.P. Boetker, S. Baldursdottir, J. Rantanen, Rheology as a tool for evaluation of melt processability of innovative dosage forms, Int. J. Pharm. 494 (2015) 623–642. https://doi.org/10.1016/j.ijpharm.2015.02.009.

[208]   T. Ponnusamy, L.B. Lawson, L.C. Freytag, D.A. Blake, R.S. Ayyala, V.T. John, In vitro degradation and release characteristics of spin coated thin films of PLGA with a "breath figure" morphology., Biomatter. 2 (2012) 77–86. https://doi.org/10.4161/biom.20390.

[209]   A.K. Mohapatra, S. Mohanty, S.K. Nayak, Effect of PEG on PLA/PEG blend and its nanocomposites: A study of thermo-mechanical and morphological characterization, Polym. Compos. 35 (2014) 283–293. https://doi.org/10.1002/pc.22660.

[210]   S. Wang, A.P. Liu, Y. Yan, T.J. Daly, N. Li, Characterization of product-related low molecular weight impurities in therapeutic monoclonal antibodies using hydrophilic interaction chromatography coupled with mass spectrometry, J. Pharm. Biomed. Anal. 154 (2018) 468–475. https://doi.org/10.1016/j.jpba.2018.03.034.

[211]   A. Melocchi, F. Parietti, A. Maroni, A. Foppoli, A. Gazzaniga, L. Zema, Hot-melt extruded filaments based on pharmaceutical grade polymers for 3D printing by fused deposition modeling, Int. J. Pharm. 509 (2016) 255–263. https://doi.org/10.1016/j.ijpharm.2016.05.036.

[212]   K. Vithani, A. Goyanes, V. Jannin, A.W. Basit, S. Gaisford, B.J. Boyd, An Overview of 3D Printing

Technologies for Soft Materials and Potential Opportunities for Lipid-based Drug Delivery Systems, Pharm. Res. 36 (2019). https://doi.org/10.1007/s11095-018-2531-1.

[213] R. Pignatello, E. Cenni, D. Micieli, C. Fotia, M. Salerno, D. Granchi, S. Avnet, M.G. Sarpietro, F. Castelli, N. Baldini, A novel biomaterial for osteotropic drug nanocarriers: Synthesis and biocompatibility evaluation of a PLGA-ALE conjugate, Nanomedicine. 4 (2009) 161–175. https://doi.org/10.2217/17435889.4.2.161.

[214] S. Shah, S. Maddineni, J. Lu, M.A. Repka, Melt extrusion with poorly soluble drugs, Int. J. Pharm. 453 (2013) 233–252. https://doi.org/10.1016/j.ijpharm.2012.11.001.

[215] C. Luebbert, F. Huxoll, G. Sadowski, G. Van Den Mooter, H. Grohganz, Amorphous-amorphous phase separation in API/polymer formulations, Molecules. 22 (2017) 296. https://doi.org/10.3390/molecules22020296.

[216] S. Ohtake, Y. Kita, T. Arakawa, Interactions of formulation excipients with proteins in solution and in the dried state, Adv. Drug Deliv. Rev. 63 (2011) 1053–1073. https://doi.org/10.1016/j.addr.2011.06.011.

[217] Y. Baek, N. Singh, A. Arunkumar, A.L. Zydney, Effects of Histidine and Sucrose on the Biophysical Properties of a Monoclonal Antibody, Pharm. Res. 34 (2017) 629–639. https://doi.org/10.1007/s11095-016-2092-0.

[218] M. Bowen, R. Turok, Y.F. Maa, Spray Drying of Monoclonal Antibodies: Investigating Powder-Based Biologic Drug Substance Bulk Storage, Dry. Technol. 31 (2013) 1441–1450. https://doi.org/10.1080/07373937.2013.796968.

[219] B. Gidwani, A. Vyas, A Comprehensive Review on Cyclodextrin-Based Carriers for Delivery of Chemotherapeutic Cytotoxic Anticancer Drugs, Biomed Res. Int. 2015 (2015). https://doi.org/10.1155/2015/198268.

[220] G. Kanojia, G.-J. Willems, H.W. Frijlink, G.F.A. Kersten, P.C. Soema, J.-P. Amorij, A Design of Experiment approach to predict product and process parameters for a spray dried influenza vaccine, Int. J. Pharm. 511 (2016) 1098–1111. https://doi.org/10.1016/J.IJPHARM.2016.08.022.

[221] M. Maury, K. Murphy, S. Kumar, A. Mauerer, G. Lee, Spray-drying of proteins: Effects of sorbitol and trehalose on aggregation and FT-IR amide I spectrum of an immunoglobulin G, Eur. J. Pharm. Biopharm. 59 (2005) 251–261. https://doi.org/10.1016/j.ejpb.2004.07.010.

[222] J.H. Cummings, A.M. Stephen, Carbohydrate terminology and classification, Eur. J. Clin. Nutr. 61 (2007) S5–S18. https://doi.org/10.1038/sj.ejcn.1602936.

[223] T.T. Do, R. Van Hooghten, G. Van den Mooter, A study of the aggregation of cyclodextrins: Determination of the critical aggregation concentration, size of aggregates and thermodynamics using isodesmic and K2–K models, Int. J. Pharm. 521 (2017) 318–326. https://doi.org/10.1016/j.ijpharm.2017.02.037.

[224] A. Dan, S. Ghosh, S.P. Moulik, Physicochemical studies on the biopolymer inulin: A critical evaluation

of its self-aggregation, aggregate-morphology, interaction with water, and thermal stability, Biopolymers. 91 (2009) 687–699. https://doi.org/10.1002/bip.21199.

[225] Y. Kim, M.N. Faqih, S.S. Wang, Factors affecting gel formation of inulin, Carbohydr. Polym. 46 (2001) 135–145. https://doi.org/10.1016/S0144-8617(00)00296-4.

[226] T.G. Barclay, C.M. Day, N. Petrovsky, S. Garg, Review of polysaccharide particle-based functional drug delivery, (2019). https://doi.org/10.1016/j.carbpol.2019.05.067.

[227] I.C. Kemp, T. Hartwig, R. Herdman, P. Hamilton, A. Bisten, S. Bermingham, Spray drying with a two-fluid nozzle to produce fine particles: Atomization, scale-up, and modeling, Dry. Technol. 34 (2016) 1243–1252. https://doi.org/10.1080/07373937.2015.1103748.

[228] N.K. Jain, I. Roy, Effect of trehalose on protein structure, Protein Sci. 18 (2009) 24–36. https://doi.org/10.1002/pro.3.

[229] T.J. Kamerzell, R. Esfandiary, S.B. Joshi, C.R. Middaugh, D.B. Volkin, Protein-excipient interactions: Mechanisms and biophysical characterization applied to protein formulation development, Adv. Drug Deliv. Rev. 63 (2011) 1118–1159. https://doi.org/10.1016/j.addr.2011.07.006.

[230] C. Nowak, J.K. Cheung, S.M. Dellatore, A. Katiyar, R. Bhat, J. Sun, G. Ponniah, A. Neill, B. Mason, A. Beck, H. Liu, J. K. Cheung, S. M. Dellatore, A. Katiyar, R. Bhat, J. Sun, G. Ponniah, A. Neill, B. Mason, A. Beck, H. Liu, Forced degradation of recombinant monoclonal antibodies: A practical guide, Taylor and Francis Inc., 2017. https://doi.org/10.1080/19420862.2017.1368602.

[231] T. Serno, R. Geidobler, G. Winter, Protein stabilization by cyclodextrins in the liquid and dried state, Adv. Drug Deliv. Rev. 63 (2011) 1086–1106. https://doi.org/10.1016/j.addr.2011.08.003.

[232] K. Rajagopal, J. Wood, B. Tran, T.W. Patapoff, T. Nivaggioli, Trehalose limits BSA aggregation in spray-dried formulations at high temperatures: Implications in preparing polymer implants for long-term protein delivery, J. Pharm. Sci. 102 (2013) 2655–2666. https://doi.org/10.1002/jps.23634.

[233] M.T. Cicerone, M.J. Pikal, K.K. Qian, Stabilization of proteins in solid form, Adv. Drug Deliv. Rev. 93 (2015) 14–24. https://doi.org/10.1016/j.addr.2015.05.006.

[234] S.F. Costa, F.M. Duarte, J.A. Covas, Thermal conditions affecting heat transfer in FDM/FFE: a contribution towards the numerical modelling of the process: This paper investigates convection, conduction and radiation phenomena in the filament deposition process, Virtual Phys. Prototyp. 10 (2015) 35–46. https://doi.org/10.1080/17452759.2014.984042.

[235] S.C. Ligon, R. Liska, J. Stampfl, M. Gurr, R. Mülhaupt, Polymers for 3D Printing and Customized Additive Manufacturing, American Chemical Society, 2017. https://doi.org/10.1021/acs.chemrev.7b00074.

[236] C. Molina, W. Kaialy, Q. Chen, D. Commandeur, A. Nokhodchi, Agglomerated novel spray-dried lactose-leucine tailored as a carrier to enhance the aerosolization performance of salbutamol sulfate from DPI formulations, (2017). https://doi.org/10.1007/s13346-017-0462-8.

[237] A. Minne, H. Boireau, M.J. Horta, R. Vanbever, Optimization of the aerosolization properties of an inhalation dry powder based on selection of excipients, Eur. J. Pharm. Biopharm. 70 (2008) 839–844. https://doi.org/10.1016/j.ejpb.2008.06.013.

[238] T. Sou, D.A. Morton, M. Williamson, E.N. Meeusen, L.M. Kaminskas, M.P. McIntosh, Spray-Dried Influenza Antigen with Trehalose and Leucine Produces an Aerosolizable Powder Vaccine Formulation that Induces Strong Systemic and Mucosal Immunity after Pulmonary Administration, J. Aerosol Med. Pulm. Drug Deliv. 28 (2015) 361–371. https://doi.org/10.1089/jamp.2014.1176.

[239] M.L. Houchin, S.A. Neuenswander, E.M. Topp, Effect of excipients on PLGA film degradation and the stability of an incorporated peptide, J. Control. Release. 117 (2007) 413–420. https://doi.org/10.1016/j.jconrel.2006.11.023.

[240] Z. Ghalanbor, M. Körber, R. Bodmeier, Interdependency of protein-release completeness and polymer degradation in PLGA-based implants, Eur. J. Pharm. Biopharm. 85 (2013) 624–630. https://doi.org/10.1016/j.ejpb.2013.03.031.

[241] A. Schädlich, S. Kempe, K. Mäder, Non-invasive in vivo characterization of microclimate pH inside in situ forming PLGA implants using multispectral fluorescence imaging, J. Control. Release. 179 (2014) 52–62. https://doi.org/10.1016/j.jconrel.2014.01.024.

[242] S. Marquette, C. Peerboom, A. Yates, L. Denis, I. Langer, K. Amighi, J. Goole, Stability study of full-length antibody (anti-TNF alpha) loaded PLGA microspheres, Int. J. Pharm. 470 (2014) 41–50. https://doi.org/10.1016/j.ijpharm.2014.04.063.

[243] D.J. Hines, D.L. Kaplan, Poly(lactic-co-glycolic) acid-controlled-release systems: experimental and modeling insights., Crit. Rev. Ther. Drug Carrier Syst. 30 (2013) 257–76. https://doi.org/10.1615/2013006475.

[244] C. Zlomke, M. Barth, K. Mäder, Polymer degradation induced drug precipitation in PLGA implants – Why less is sometimes more, Eur. J. Pharm. Biopharm. 139 (2019) 142–152. https://doi.org/10.1016/j.ejpb.2019.03.016.

[245] J. Hermosilla, R. Pérez-Robles, A. Salmerón-García, S. Casares, J. Cabeza, J. Bones, N. Navas, Comprehensive biophysical and functional study of ziv-aflibercept: characterization and forced degradation, Sci. Rep. 10 (2020). https://doi.org/10.1038/s41598-020-59465-7.

[246] Y. Hu, M. Rogunova, V. Topolkaraev, A. Hiltner, E. Baer, Aging of poly(lactide)/poly(ethylene glycol) blends. Part 1. Poly(lactide) with low stereoregularity, Polymer (Guildf). 44 (2003) 5701–5710. https://doi.org/10.1016/S0032-3861(03)00614-1.

[247] J.R. White, Polymer ageing: physics, chemistry or engineering? Time to reflect, Comptes Rendus Chim. 9 (2006) 1396–1408. https://doi.org/10.1016/j.crci.2006.07.008.

[248] M. Ovacik, K. Lin, Tutorial on Monoclonal Antibody Pharmacokinetics and Its Considerations in Early Development, Clin. Transl. Sci. 11 (2018) 540–552. https://doi.org/10.1111/cts.12567.

[249] K.T. Xenaki, S. Oliveira, P.M.P. van Bergen en Henegouwen, Antibody or antibody fragments: Implications for molecular imaging and targeted therapy of solid tumors, Front. Immunol. 8 (2017) 1287. https://doi.org/10.3389/fimmu.2017.01287.

[250] D. Schweizer, T. Serno, A. Goepferich, Controlled release of therapeutic antibody formats, Eur. J. Pharm. Biopharm. 88 (2014) 291–309. https://doi.org/10.1016/J.EJPB.2014.08.001.

[251] W.K. Redekop, D. Mladsi, The Faces of Personalized Medicine: A Framework for Understanding Its Meaning and Scope, Value Heal. 16 (2013) S4. https://doi.org/10.1016/j.jval.2013.06.005.

APPENDIX

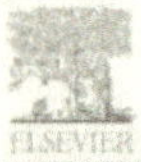

Contents lists available at ScienceDirect

International Journal of Pharmaceutics

journal homepage: www.elsevier.com/locate/ijpharm

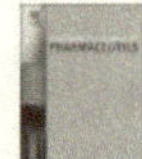

Investigation of the parameters used in fused deposition modeling of poly (lactic acid) to optimize 3D printing sessions

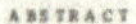

E. Carlier[a,*], S. Marquette[b], C. Peerboom[b], L. Denis[b], S. Benali[c], J-M. Raquez[c], K. Amighi[a], J. Goole[a]

[a] Laboratory of Pharmaceutics and Biopharmaceutics, Université libre de Bruxelles, Faculty of Pharmacy, Brussels 1050, Belgium
[b] Laboratory UCB Pharma, Biological Formulation Development Group, Braine-l'Alleud, Belgium
[c] Laboratory of Polymers and Composite Materials, IMOMS, Mons, Belgium

ARTICLE INFO

Keywords:
3D printing
Fused deposition modeling
Thermomechanical properties
Printing parameters
Poly(lactic acid)

ABSTRACT

This study assesses the feasibility of printing implantable devices using 3D printing Fused deposition modeling (FDM) technology. The influence of the deposition temperature, the deposition rate and the layer thickness on the printing process and the physical properties of the devices were evaluated. The filaments were composed of neat poly(lactic acid) (PLA) and blends of different plasticizers (polyethylene glycol 400 (PEG 400), triacetine (TA), acetyltriethyl citrate (ATEC) and triethyl citrate (TEC)) at 10% (w/w). The assessment of thermo-mechanical characterization and morphology of both filaments and devices (cylinders and dog bones) were performed. The influence of each parameter was evaluated using a design of experiment (DoE) and the significance of the results was discussed. A large amount of data about the evaluation of FDM process parameters are already available in the literature. However, specific insights needed to be increased into the impact of the use of PLA and plasticized PLA raw material on the feasibility of printing devices in three dimensions. To conclude, the ductility was improved with a high layer thickness, low temperature and using ATEC. Whereas, adhesion was promoted with an increase in temperature, a lower layer thickness and adding TA.

1. Introduction

Fused deposition modeling (FDM) is a type of additive manufacturing technology that allows the production of three-dimensional (3D) devices from a computer-aided design (CAD) file (Carneiro et al., 2015; Jin et al., 2015). FDM is an user-friendly, adaptable, low-cost technique to quickly print prototypes with complex geometry (Kantaros and Karalekas, 2013; Panda et al., 2017). However, the FDM technique is characterized by some limitations due to its use of high temperatures. These temperatures may lead to potential thermal degradation, shrinkage issues, low surface quality and poor resolution. Such issues drastically limit the number of thermoplastic polymers that can be used, as well as the mixture of these with plasticizers when a decrease in their glass transition temperature (T_g) is needed to reduce the printing temperature (Allman et al., 2016; Bhushan and Caspers, 2017).

Moreover, although FDM is a fairly well-known 3DP technique, it is still a complex process to understand and control. This complexity is due to the relatively high number of parameters that may be modulated as well as their interdependence on the physiochemical properties of the final printed device. As these parameters are set during the design step (pre-processing) and remain constant throughout the printing process, it is still difficult to determine the appropriate parameters to obtain the desired rendering (Mohamed et al., 2016). Several studies have focused on the optimization of the FDM process parameters, including mechanical properties and the anisotropic behaviour of thermoplastic materials during their extrusion through the nozzle (Allyson et al., 2016; Croccolo et al., 2013; Tymrak et al., 2014). Indeed, previous works have demonstrated that tensile parameters such as build

Abbreviations: X_c, degree of crystallinity; 3DP, three-dimensional printing; ABS, acrylonitrile butadiene styrene; ASTM, American Society for Testing and Materials; ATEC, acetyltriethyl citrate; CAD, computer-aided design; DoE, design of experiment; DSC, differential scanning calorimetry; EVA, ethylene vinyl acetate; FDM, fused deposition modeling; HME, hot melt extrusion; MFI, melt flow index; MPa, megapascal; Mw, molecular weight; PCL, poly(ε-caprolactone); PEG 400, polyethylene glycol 400; PLA, poly(lactic acid); PVA, polyvinyl alcohol; RP, rapid prototyping; rpm, revolutions per minute; SEM, scanning electron microscopy; SSE, single screw extruder; TA, triacetin; TEC, triethyl citrate; T_c, crystallization temperature; T_g, glass transition temperature; TGA, thermogravimetric analysis; Tm, melting temperature; % (w/w), weight percentage

* Corresponding author.
E-mail address: emicie.carlier@ulb.ac.be (E. Carlier).

https://doi.org/10.1016/j.ijpharm.2019.05.008
Received 10 February 2019; Received in revised form 5 April 2019; Accepted 4 May 2019
Available online 06 May 2019

Contents lists available at ScienceDirect

International Journal of Pharmaceutics

journal homepage: www.elsevier.com/locate/ijpharm

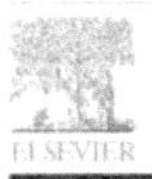

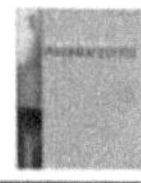

Development of mAb-loaded 3D-printed (FDM) implantable devices based on PLGA

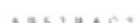

E. Carlier[a,*], S. Marquette[b], C. Peerboom[b], K. Amighi[a], J. Goole[a]

[a] Laboratory of Pharmaceutics and Biopharmaceutics, Université libre de Bruxelles, Faculty of Pharmacy, 1050 Brussels, Belgium
[b] Department of Biological Pharmaceutical Sciences, UCB Pharma S.A., 1420 Braine-l'Alleud, Belgium

ARTICLE INFO

Keywords:
3D printing
Monoclonal antibody
Fused deposition modelling
Implantable systems

ABSTRACT

The main objective of this work was to explore the feasibility to print monoclonal antibody (mAb)-loaded implantable systems using fused-deposition modelling (FDM) to build complex dosage form designs. Indeed, to our knowledge, this work is the first investigation of mAb-loaded devices using FDM. To make this possible, different steps were developed and optimized. A mAb solution was stabilized using trehalose (TRE), sucrose (SUC), hydroxypropyl-β-cyclodextrin (HP-β-CD), sorbitol or inulin (INU) in order to be spray dried (SD). Printable filaments were then made of poly(lactide-co-glycolide) (PLGA) and mAb powder (15% w/w) using hot melt extrusion (HME). The FDM process was optimized to print these filaments without altering the mAb stability. TRE was selected and associated to L-leucine (LEU) to increase the mAb stability. The stability was then evaluated considering high and low molecular weight species levels. The mAb-based devices were well-stabilized with the selected excipients during both the HME and the FDM processes. The 3D-printed devices showed sustained-release profiles with a low burst effect. The mAb-binding capacity was preserved up to 70% following the whole fabrication process. These promising results demonstrate that FDM could be used to produce mAb-loaded devices with good stability, affinity and sustained-release profiles of the mAb.

1. Introduction

Fused-deposition modelling (FDM), a 3D printing (3DP) process, is currently an integral part of the pharmaceutical field (Azad et al., 2020). This technology is an extrusion-based 3DP method that uses heat to melt a thermoplastic polymer filament to build an object in a layer-wise manner. The use of 3DP allows the production of any kind of shape, starting from a digital design (Norman et al., 2017). The emergence of FDM as the most investigated technique for printing drug-delivery systems (DDS) is attributed to its high flexibility, the low cost of the printers and its ability to produce hollow objects (Alhnan et al., 2016; Azad et al., 2020). Moreover, the ability of 3DP to complement mass production techniques could be interesting to develop specific DDS in small batches with tailored doses for personalized medicine (Sadia et al., 2020). The main drawback remains the lack of pharmaceutical-grade polymers available to be used in FDM.

However, FDA-approved grade polymers for human use, such as poly (lactic acid) (PLA) and polyvinyl alcohol (PVA), are commonly used as thermoplastic polymers that may be used to make drug-loaded printable filaments (Jamróz et al., 2018). Therefore, numerous academic research efforts have focused on the development of polymeric filaments loaded with different active pharmaceutical ingredients (APIs). Hot melt extrusion (HME) is already widely described, and implemented in the pharmaceutical field to produce such drug-loaded printable filaments (Goyanes et al., 2015b).

HME is based on the melting of polymeric material that is extruded through a die to obtain a homogeneous drug-loaded filament. HME is a solvent-free process that may easily be scaled up (Tiwari et al., 2016). However, this technique is based on the use of relatively high temperatures, which may usually be reduced by adding a plasticizer to decrease the glass transition temperature (T_g) of the polymer. Another alternative to decrease the extrusion temperature could be the use of thermoplastic polymers characterized by a low molecular weight (Prudenberg et al., 2011). Moreover, HME has already been investigated to develop protein-based formulations that were characterized by a controlled release of the loaded API over time (Cosse et al., 2016; Duque et al., 2018; Ghalanbor et al., 2010). Indeed, sustained release allows the number of administrations to be reduced to improve patient compliance as well as to ensure the therapeutic efficacy (Anwall and Anglian-strong, 2018). Poly(lactide-co-glycolide) (PLGA) has been widely investigated and is already a well-known pharmaceutical-grade

* Corresponding author.
E-mail address: estcerrie.carlier@ulb.be (E. Carlier).

https://doi.org/10.1016/j.ijpharm.2021.120337
Received 15 December 2020; Received in revised form 25 January 2021; Accepted 30 January 2021
Available online 4 February 2021
0378-5173/© 2021 Published by Elsevier B.V.